Living Balanced

Healthy Mind & Body
Reference Guide

Stacey A. Kimbrell

W we should "Eat to live, not live to eat." We need to improve our health by changing poor diet habits to healthy ones. In America, this can be difficult, but with much prayer and the determination to have a healthy and happy family, anything is possible! You will find that I am a believer in Christ. He has given me strength, courage, understanding and knowledge. For that I will be forever grateful. Please hear this... *You are responsible for your actions!* Whether old or young, you are in charge of your future and can change things for the better! Get excited for yourself! Don't look to others for approval, and don't let others control your feelings and bring you down. Live your life boldly with confidence and self-esteem! Take pride in ALL you do! No matter what your beliefs, this book will guide you towards becoming a happier and healthier person.

"Do you not know that you are the temple of God and that the Spirit of God dwells in you?" (1 Corinthians 3:16)

"...Through Christ (and His strength), we can do all things". Phil. 4:13
"...the fruit thereof shall be for meat, and the leaf thereof for medicine". (Ezekiel 47:12)
"Whatever you do whether you eat or drink, do unto the glory of God." (1 Cor. 10:31)
"...The leaves of the tree are for the healing of the nations". Revelation 22:2

"The Lord spoke unto Moses saying: "Take thou also unto thee principal spices of pure myrrh...of sweet cinnamon...of sweet calamus...of cassia...and of olive...and thou shalt make it an oil of holy ointment, an ointment compound after the art of the apothecary"... (Exodus 30:22-25)

"Be very careful, then, how you live - not as unwise but as wise, making the most of every opportunity, because the days are evil. Therefore do not be foolish, but understand what the Lord's will is. Always giving thanks to God the Father for everything, in the name of our Lord Jesus Christ." (Ephesians 5: 15-20)

Finally, "Be strong in the Lord and in his mighty power; "Put on the full armor of God so that you can take your stand against the devil's schemes". (Ephesians 6:11)

LivingAnointed.com is available to you.
You can receive a monthly email health bulletin, our website will give more information on health and wellness, recipes, health videos, local events, information and links to many different services and health related topics. E-mail me for a FREE copy of the *Missing Link CD.*

Disclaimer: It is not the intention of *Living Balanced* to provide specific medical advice, but rather to share research and experience. *Living Balanced* hopes you may better understand your health and any challenges, from a more natural perspective. *Living Balanced* encourages you to make your own health care decisions based upon your research and in partnership with a qualified health care professional.

Dedication

I dedicate this book first to Jesus Christ, because without Him nothing is possible. He has given me the strength, faith, ability, discernment, understanding, knowledge, and open mind to learn all I have in such a short time. All praises be to Christ! "For you were bought at a price; therefore glorify God in your body, and in your spirit, which are God's" (1 Corinthians 6:20).

Steve, I thank God everyday for such a wonderful husband who happens to be my knight in shining armor here on earth. You have taught me so much over our years together, through love, patience, understanding, commitment, a willingness to change and lead our family in honoring God. Thank you for supporting me!

My boys August & Austin! You love me despite my faults and continue to bless me with love and understanding when I am serving others. Also, you have done a great job being open-minded and changing your food choices to healthier ones. You have surpassed my expectation in our new lifestyle and for that I am grateful.

August, you are growing quick, 6' and 16 years old. Being the oldest is not easy and changing your lifestyle at this age can be difficult. You have done extraordinarily well under these circumstances. I applaud you for taking a stand in what you believe in and pray you continue. You are a very special young man and I am pleased that God has given you to me.

Austin, at your tender age of 12, you amaze me! Your interest and compassion for helping others is an honor to me. Keep up the good work with your science fair experiments. I believe that you have God given knowledge, mercy, compassion and insight to help educate and heal people. I can't wait to see what the Lord has in store for you. You are very special and I Love You!

Dear Readers, what a great opportunity this is for you to learn. Explore and share with yourself, friends, and family. Please understand, it is YOUR job to take care of YOURSELF first, then you can help others.

If you have children, you have a greater responsibility to raise your children in a loving, caring, respectful, and healthy environment. We are our children's future! How we teach, mold, and love our children will determine what type of adults they will become.

Our Mind is very powerful! Learn how to control it!

Contents

Acknowledgments

Dr. G. Young, *thank you for all of your hard work, dedication and determination.*

Dr. Nathan Peachey *has been a gift from God for me. From the first day I met him, he has been willing to teach me everything from A-Z. I will forever be grateful for the knowledge he holds and has shared with me unselfishly.*

Without **Barb Morse** *I may never have found out how to heal my body naturally. Through her, I have learned how to rely on God, become a better wife, mother, and person.*

My mom, Heidi, *has inspired me in her courage to get off all of her medications and learn how to handle life in an entirely new healthy way. Medication free since Nov. 17, 2008 and you are still doing well! She has made tremendous leaps in faith and health. Way to go Mom!*

Ruth Dec *has inspired me and taught me how God sees us and about His will for us to be healthy here on earth. You have given and shared all you have in compassion, time, goods, services, money, and love. You are a true blessing to this world and our life.*

Nique Beer *has really taken an initiative to learn a new way of approaching health and nutrition with herself and daughters Jenee and Maria. I am blessed to have Nique as a friend and love seeing her strive to improve the health and well being of others.*

Sandy Flenniken, *what a giver and a teacher! I love you woman and would do anything for you. You are a great inspiration!*

Grandma Ashby, Lovella, *I love you. Your unconditional love is amazing. Your willingness to make changes at this stage in your life is so encouraging to me and others. Thank you for all of the love and support you have given me. Grandpa would be proud of you!*

Tina Serra, *I am truly privileged that God has brought you and your family into my life. Thank you for your guidance, perseverance and dedication to help me recognize my priorities.*

Shannon Hudson, *truly gave me HOPE that, through Young Living Essential Oils, I could heal or treat my bladder disease for the first time in my life, without any more surgeries.*

Karen Malone *truly has a gift from God to serve, care, and love on people no matter who you are, where you are, where you have been or what you have done. Your neverending energy makes me wonder sometimes if you are really human.*

Sue Jaster, *you have inspired me to become a better mother. Your dedication to Christ, your husband and children is remarkable and uplifting and I aspire to be more like you.*

Introduction

August 1, 2007, is the year our HOPE was restored and the time my family took our first step toward improving our health habits! If you would have told me my children would eat a carrot on their own, turn away from Hawaiian punch, my incurable bladder disease (interstitial cystitis) would be cured or I would be able to read well, I would not have believed you. I would have likely said, "Yeah, right!" The year that I turned forty was simultaneously the hardest, yet most rewarding year of my life. The amazingly short amount of time it took for our family's health and emotional turn around was one of the multiple miracles I have witnessed. Our bodies (myself, Steve my husband since 1994, and our sons August -13 and Austin - 9) are now disease and illness free. We are finally able to think and lovingly communicate clearly. We had no idea, or ever considered the dangerous chemicals in our foods, drinks or skin care or how they affected our temper, behavior, and health. Without neurotoxins clogging our brains, we are now able to think clearly. We are able to stop and rationalize before reacting. Previously there was yelling and anger, now there are words spoken in love and kindness towards one another. I'm excited! I hope that my family's story can encourage you to take the first steps towards healing and restoration of your body, mind, and spirit.

We noticed a difference in just a few weeks. Hope literally turned into reality for the Kimbrell family. Camping in the woods, this chance encounter became one of the best moments in my life. By reading "Living Balanced" you will explore many different ways to heal your body and restore your health. It doesn't matter where you live or your income level, there are things you can do to improve your health. In the last year we have made a 180-degree turnaround. We took back or threw away all of our toxic chemicals, changed our diet to whole food nutrition, started drinking healthy juices, and consumed healthy sources of vitamins, herbs, and oils. The Kimbrell bodies have been restored! We came off all prescription and over the counter medication. We've been healed of dermatitis, eyesight issues (my glasses), long healing recovery, chronic sinusitis, allergies, depression, constipation, lung infections, dyslexia, ADHD (my son's learning disabilities) staphylococcus infections, cellulites, hemorrhoids, bad attitudes and tempers.

The two major struggles in my life had been dyslexia and interstitial cystitis (IC); keeping me from writing, accounting, and even reading to name a few of the things I'd always wanted to do. I am not ashamed to admit that I had never read a complete book until September of 2007. This is my reason for such excitement. My husband Steve, the love of my life, is in awe of my new abilities. My interstitial cystitis is no longer an issue. I had been taking antibiotics for seventeen years, urinating 30 to 60 times a day with blood and tissue. I endured chronic yeast (candida) infections and had many surgeries and procedures done in an attempt to repair my IC. As a result of taking so many prescribed medications, I am now resistant to all antibiotics. At a health seminar in July of 2007, I was introduced to a fruit drink containing lycium barbarum (wolfberry) and its healing powers. We were skeptical at first, although hopeful because of desperation and lack of knowledge. We listened to the suggestions at the seminar and decided to give it a try. Two years after seemingly overdosing on the fruit drink NingXia Red (6 oz a day for one month), I started to see great changes in my family, so much for the better I began to research during all my free time. *Living Balanced, Healthy Mind & Body Reference Guide* is the compilation of my research. I travel, teach, and consult on health, wellness and chemical awareness and I am cured of my interstitial cystitis.

Having worked in the medical field for thirteen years, I have knowledge of the body and how it functions. I was taught to give the patient temporary relief by dealing with the symptoms. I now look at the root cause of a problem. Your body will automatically start to correct itself when you deal with the cause of your health issue and not the symptoms. Thanks to that seminar on healthy living, I have officially dedicated my life to the ministry of educating people who want to heal and/or restore their body to a healthy, pain free, synthetic drug free way of life. My new goal is to continue in this field and be in a place to help others to do the same.

With what I now know, I hate to hear the statements, "I'll change after I finish my six bottles of Kaboom," or "I just bought a pack of Crystal Light." You can go return them! I did, over $150 worth of products with no receipt. It can be done. If some of the items are non-returnable, then throw them away. Why would you want to poison yourself one more day? Who is in charge of your life? YOU! Will it be hard at first to make changes? Most assuredly, yes! Will you like it right off the bat? You probably won't. Will you have slip-ups along the way while you learn? You probably will. The real question is, "Can you do it?" Yes, of course you can! I want to help anyone who truly wants to make a commitment to change his or her life!

One common food example for the American family is french (American) fries. When we found out how bad french fries are, we had to make a decision! We had the choice to continue on the path of chronic illness or change our life style from the Standard American Diet (SAD) to a whole food nutrition lifestyle. It is these little life changes that will help you heal. Knowing it would not be easy, we prayed for God's help and guidance. We had always taught our children, August and Austin, to rely on the Lord for all things. Yet, we hadn't when it came to our health and diet habits.

Whatever your spiritual belief, it can play a large role in your recovery. The secret of my family's success is asking God for mercy and grace to change our taste buds, so we could enjoy the foods that please Him and heal our bodies.

I am a Biblically based health advocate, believing our bodies are the temple and we need to treat it as such. "Whatever you eat or drink or whatever you do, do all for the glory of God" (1 Corinthians 10:31). "My people are destroyed for lack of knowledge" (Hosea 4:6). Notice it is not a lack of prayer, nor lack of faith, or lack of love, but for a "lack of knowledge"! This is deep! If you really think about it, everything that is wrong with the world today stems from a lack of knowledge! The key to success in anything is always some form of education, knowledge, or wisdom.

The hardest part of my job now is trying to help those who don't love or respect themselves. We should take responsibility and respect ourselves. This is the best thing you can do if you have children. It will teach them to do the same. Children will model your actions. Create a positive, health conscious environment so they will grow up with a healthy amount of self-esteem, confidence and knowledge of who they are and what they represent.

People often say to me "God blesses my food no matter what it is." I disagree! How can God bless food that doesn't mold and is full of synthetic or toxic chemicals that He never intended for us to consume? The purpose of a blessing is to give assistance where it is needed. With fake, synthetic, processed foods they need no blessing, they need a miracle to change into something healthy. It already has a shelf life of 5 to 1,000 times longer than real, natural foods. Don't believe me? How long will a cake made from scratch last? A few days, maybe a week. Now, what about a Twinkie? With all the processing and preservatives, it could last two to three years. Our society is not getting any healthier, so you will have to retrain your brain. America spends the most on health care among the largest nations, yet we are the most health-troubled nation in the world. America also produces and consumes the most diet products in the world, yet we continue to widen the gap on the rest of the world with our widening waistlines. It's not rocket science! Something is wrong with this picture! It does not matter what your spiritual belief is. Once you hear the truth, you are then accountable for it. I don't even want you to take my word for this. Go and research it for yourself so you will know the truth!

I will tell you up front that this book is going to point out some of the bad things you have been doing unknowingly. The foods you use, the way you prepare certain foods, some of the products you use, maybe even some of the staples your family currently depends on. At the same time, it will show you how to change things to help improve your health and life. Some people fear change. I personally love change! If I can find a way to improve my family, my community, and myself I will strive to do so.

Please don't worry about getting overwhelmed. Take baby steps. First think about your life right now. Can it be improved? If so, then read this book. What do you have to lose? You likely have more to gain than you have to lose. Education is the key! Once you read it, just start making some of the necessary changes to move forward, then make some more. In a month or two, you can be on your way to a whole new body, mind and spirit! I have seen it happen so many times. It happened to me!

Warning: You will likely be upset when you find out the actions of big business, manufacturers and sometimes even the government. Some things they have either allowed to happen or made happen to the public, simply out of greed. From my experience, anger is not going to help you. I think, at times, I have been mad enough for all of us. Don't waste your time in anger; it will only slow down your healing process.

I wish you much success and many blessings in your journey to a new, happy and healthier you! Remember the three easy steps!

Step 1   Pray for strength and courage to act on your new knowledge.
Step 2   Get rid of the toxic chemicals that we use and consume everyday.
Step 3   Begin to use natural methods of healing your body to restore and maintain your health.

Update 2011, We are still drug/medication free! We have not had bad fast food in 3.5 years and we just celebrated our 4 year anniversary of learning about the oils and health.

August, 16 and Austin, 12 are still doing great. Infact, they help educate others on how to live a healthier lifestyle. We just recently team taught at a health conference. August spoke on 1st Aid with Essential Oils and how to make healthy foods taste yummy. August does most of the cooking in the home and you will see the drawing he created for me in the book - "The Tree Of Life". I just love it! Austin teaches on MSG and neurotoxins, why french fries don't mold, and how to do the liver stone cleanse.

Blessings,
Stacey
8/2011

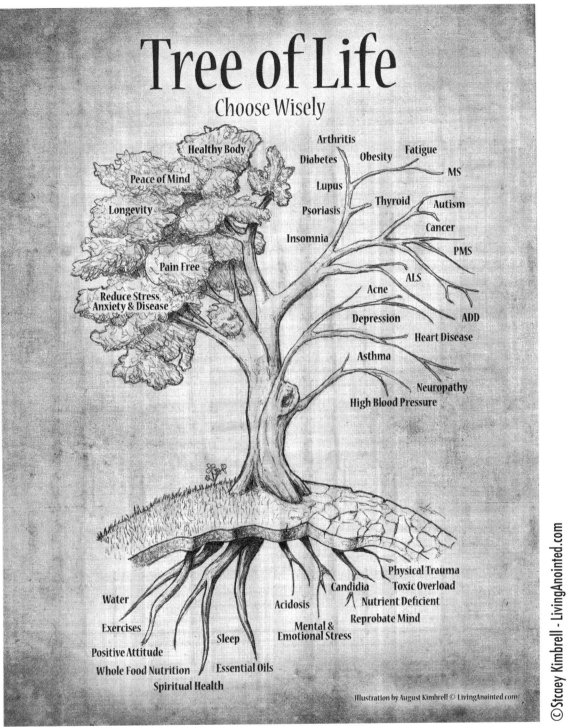

Tree of Life
Choose Wisely

Healthy Body
Peace of Mind
Longevity
Pain Free
Reduce Stress, Anxiety & Disease

Arthritis
Diabetes
Obesity
Fatigue
MS
Lupus
Thyroid
Autism
Psoriasis
Cancer
Insomnia
PMS
ALS
Acne
Depression
ADD
Heart Disease
Asthma
Neuropathy
High Blood Pressure

Physical Trauma
Toxic Overload
Candidia
Nutrient Deficient
Acidosis
Reprobate Mind
Water
Exercises
Mental & Emotional Stress
Sleep
Positive Attitude
Whole Food Nutrition
Essential Oils
Spiritual Health

Illustration by August Kimbrell © LivingAnointed.com

©Stcaey Kimbrell - LivingAnointed.com

The "Tree of Life" is a choice! Choose wisely! I love this! It was drawn by my son August at the age of 15. On the right the roots (foundation) are not deep or healthy. This is where illnesses and diseases starts. The ground is dehydrated and cracked. In the trunk there is a person who is weak and sick. On the left, the roots are deep and strong. The soil is nourished. Within the trunk is a person flourishing with a healthy state of Mind, Body and Spirit!

THE CAUSE

O ur health and the health of our family is one of our greatest responsibilities in life. I see the failure to accurately assess "potential danger" keeping people locked in all kinds of unhealthy situations, such as stress, unhappiness, a constant state of frustration, poor eating and exercise habits (lifestyle), and hurtful relationships, all of which result in overall poor health. This reference book will guide you in making positive changes to improve your health and well-being. It is important to have an open mind and pray that God will show you the truth.

IMPROVE YOUR HEALTH AND WELL-BEING NATURALLY

My story began in July of 2007. We were camping up North in Michigan at Rose Hill Resort when my son August twisted his ankle playing flashlight tag. I carried him on my back to the main cabin and asked the owner, Barb, if she had any Motrin for him. She said, "No, we use natural medicine called Young Living Essential Oils. I said, "Ok, I'll try that." So Barb rubbed the oils on his ankle and about five minutes later he got up and ran off. I couldn't believe it! I instantly wanted to know more. She invited us to attend a class about health and nutrition the next evening. So, Saturday came and all six of us went. Steve, Grandma Ashby and I were amazed at the stories of healing. This gave us hope for my bladder disease, interstitial cystitis (IC).

The teacher, Shannon Hudson, had made a statement about how bad toothpaste is. I thought she was exaggerating and a little "off her rocker." Now remember, we're camping, so when I got back to the cabin, I looked at our toothpaste and began to read the tube. I was

> If you only take one thing to heart from this book, let it be the challenge to start reading the ingredients on the labels on all of your products.

shocked to see that the container said, *"If you accidentally swallow, seek professional help or contact a poison control center immediately."* When I got home from camping the next day, I began a Google search on each ingredient found in toothpaste. The following is what I found one tube of toothpaste can contain: Alcohol, SD Alcohol, artificial flavoring, artificial food dyes and colors, Aspartame, Carrageenin, Chlorhexidine, Poloxmer 403, Sodium Hydroxide (Lye), Synthetic Glycerine, Fluoride, PEG-32, Pentasodium triphosphate, Benzoic Acid, Polysorbate 80, Propylene glycol, Saccharin, Silica, Sodium lauryl sulfate (SLS), Sodium monofluorophosphate, Sucralose® (Splenda®), Tetrasodium pyrophosphate, Titanium dioxide, and Triclosan. **All are toxic ingredients and can cause disruption of our endocrine system; organ system toxicity, cancer, and harsh irritation to the skin. Our brain and nervous system can be impacted at low doses.** Mind you, this is for adult and children's toothpaste and mouthwash.

I then went through EVERY food item, medication, hair and skin care product, plastic container, and cleaning product in my home. I continued to do a Google search or MSDS (Material Safety Data Sheet) on every ingredient. I was not pleased to have been misled and to be ignorant of what I was using, eating, and giving to my family. I have made it my goal to let people know what a difference it can make to be *FREE* of all these toxic chemicals. I can truly say that since my house has been free of MSG, aspartame, food dyes, high fructose corn syrup, and toxic chemicals in our skin care and cleaning products, my family's health, attitudes, and behavior have done a 180-degree turn for the better. I pray you will seek the truth, be open to it, and then have the willpower and determination to make positive, healthy changes in your life.

One of the most important aspects of living a healthy and prosperous life is to understand "potential dangers." By this I mean, are we really aware of the risk we are taking daily when we **use** or **eat** toxic chemicals/poisons? Have you ever thought about how it affects your health? Too often, with our busy lifestyles, we don't read our labels or question the ingredients, resulting in our making decisions based on incomplete or inaccurate information. This is a huge mistake with significant consequences! For example, did you know that MSG, soy and propylene glycol (antifreeze) are in some baby formulas, not to mention hydrogenated and genetically modified oils? Propylene glycol is the main ingredient in the solution that we drink (Go Lightly and Miralax) before we have a colonoscopy and that it is in toothpaste, frosting, cake mixes, Slim-fast, toaster breakfast pastries and even skin care. MSG actually has over twenty different names, and it is in everything from chips, to soup (at least three levels per can), seasoning packets, and skin care.

Are you familiar with soy? There is increasing research on the negative health effects of soy and soybeans: cancer, heart disease, osteoporosis, brain atrophy, endocrine system disorders including the thyroid and infertility, heart and blood clotting. Soybeans are high in phytic acid, present in the bran or hulls of all seeds. It's a substance that can block the uptake of essential minerals - calcium, magnesium, copper, iron and especially zinc - in the intestinal tract.

Something to think about

Aspartame is the technical name for the artificial sweetener used in Nutrasweet, 951, Ajinomoto, Equal, Splenda, Sucralose and many other brand names. It has been linked to many health issues. It is unbelievable that the FDA even allowed on the market. It can be found in ice cream, soda, yogurt, milk, cookies, bread, vitamins, prescriptions, and vaccines. Why is it used in our vaccines? Do our veins care if it tastes sweet or not, or are they just trying to poison us? These sweetners break down our immune system, leaving us vulnerable to sickness and disease.

There are recent reports on toxic levels of lead in lipstick, toys, and bad batches of vaccines given to our babies (Good Morning America, CNN, and 20/20). There are toxic levels of Bisphenol-A found in baby bottles and all plastic containers with the numbers 3, 6, and 7 on the bottom. I find it interesting how all of the multi-symptom flu and cold medications for children have been pulled off the shelves recently. All of this seriously affects our health and future whether we are young or old.

When is the last time we went to the doctor with an ailment and the physician said, "Let's find out why you are feeling this way," instead of just giving you medication to cover up the symptoms?

Here is a true story that happened to my family. In June of 2007 my husband and I took our eight year old son to his pediatrician because he had warts popping up everywhere. I had told my son that he needed to start eating better foods. When we got to the doctor, my son asked him if eating better food would keep his body healthier. To our shock the pediatrician said, "Food has no bearing on our health." We couldn't believe it!

Upon further research, I learned that warts and cold sores occur when our immune system is low. Our body should be able to fight these ailments off easily. Please know that I am not against medical doctors. We do need them and benefit from their expertise and training. However, many have received little or no schooling on the benefits and importance of health in relation to food and proper nutrition.

Almost eighteen billion dollars are spent on skin and body care products each year in America, with the hope that they will make you look and feel younger. **Most of these products contain chemicals that may be hazardous to our health and make us age quicker.** Humans are very vulnerable to chemicals because the skin is extremely porous. Cosmetic and body care product ingredients are absorbed through the skin, penetrating in significant amounts when left on for long periods. Many are carcinogenic, mimic estrogen, containing lead, formaldehyde, and pesticides, including DDT etc.

I believe if we can't consume a product such as toothpaste, lotion, cream, eye drops, essential oils etc. we shouldn't put it on our skin or inhale it. Remember, **if it is toxic when taken orally, it is toxic when applied topically or inhaled.**

See "Take Complete Control of Your Health"
Clifford, Catherine. (2008). one in 3 toys is toxic
CNNMoney; http://money.cnn.com/2008/12/03/news/companies/toxic_toys/index.htm

Are You Going To Eat That?
How America is Tricked by Big Business

The ingredient lists on food products are designed to inform consumers about the contents in the product. The reality is that these lists are used by food manufacturers and designed to deceive consumers and trick them into thinking that products are healthier (or of a better quality) than they really are. Our biggest mistake is in trusting the government to ensure the safety of our food. Rarely will a product be deemed unfit for human consumption until it is determined beyond a reasonable doubt to be dangerous. It can take generations to determine if a food additive is harmful. There are over 2000 Government approved non-food additives. You are the only people you can hold accountable for what you eat. The government is a business that excels in *marketing*. **Food Manufacturers actually "buy" shelf space and positions at grocery stores.** That is why the most profitable foods, the ones with the lowest quality ingredients, are the most visible on aisle end caps, checkout lanes, and eye-level shelves throughout the store.

TRICKS OF THE FOOD TRADE: DECEIVING CONSUMERS

If the Nutrition Facts section on food packaging lists all the substances that go into a food product, how can they deceive consumers? Here are a few of the most common ways:

Most people *do not read* the ingredient lists of the foods they buy. Labels are designed to entice you to buy the product. The first three ingredients on the list are about 85% of the total product by weight. Those ingredients need to be the best ingredients. Let's look at wheat flour. It can say wheat on the label and not be whole wheat. It must say **whole wheat or 100% whole wheat or stone ground** in the ingredients list. It can even say 100% wheat on the label, but that only means it does contain some 100% wheat, not that the product is made entirely of pure whole wheat.

Another common trick is to **distribute sugars among many ingredients**, so they don't appear in the top three. For example, a manufacturer may use a combination of sucrose, high-fructose corn syrup, corn syrup solids, brown sugar, dextrose and other sugar ingredients to make sure none of them are present in large enough quantities to attain a top position on the ingredients lists. Remember, ingredients are listed in order of their proportion in the food. This fools consumers into thinking the food product isn't really made mostly of sugar, while in reality it is. It is a way to shift sugar farther down the ingredients list, thereby misinforming consumers about the sugar content of the whole product.

"Label padding" means to **pad the list with miniscule amounts of great-sounding ingredients.** You see this in personal care products like shampoo. Companies claim to offer "herbal" shampoos that have practically no detectable levels of real herbs in them. In food, companies pad the ingredient lists with healthy-sounding "berries," "herbs" or "super foods" that are often only present in miniscule amounts.

HIDING DANGEROUS INGREDIENTS

Hiding dangerous ingredients behind innocent-sounding names is a common packaging technique to fool consumers into thinking they are safe. The highly carcinogenic ingredient, sodium nitrite, for example, sounds perfectly innocent. However it is well documented that sodium nitrite causes brain tumors, pancreatic cancer, colon cancer and many other cancers (search Google Scholar for sodium nitrite).

Carmine sounds like an innocent food coloring, but it is actually made from the smashed bodies of red cochineal beetles. Of course, no one would eat strawberry yogurt if it said, "insect-based red food coloring" on the label.

Ingesting high levels of MSG (mono-sodium glutamate) and artificial sweeteners is the biggest health mistake that people make because these additives contain high quantities of excitotoxins. An excitotoxin makes your brain think something tastes good when it doesn't. An excitotoxin causes your brain nerves to fire so quickly that they actually get burned out. Excitotoxins kill brain cells. Two well-known excitotoxins are MSG and aspartame. They both kill brain cells in everyone, but those who say that they are allergic to MSG are just more sensitive. The first sign of an excitotoxin is a headache. Excitotoxins are damaging our nervous systems and causing untold health problems. They are added to thousands of foods and grocery products through a dozen different innocent-sounding ingredients. They cause imbalances in the endocrine system function, disable normal appetite regulation and cause consumers to keep eating more food, thus contributing to nationwide obesity. MSG is mostly used as a flavor enhancer, which heightens the taste of foods. This heightened experience can create an addiction to the chemical. **MSG has 20+ names and is routinely hidden in foods with these ingredient names:** yeast extract, torula yeast, hydrolyzed and autolyzed (anything).

See Dr. Colbert, MD "Eat this and Live" pg 30
See "MSG The Excitotoxin"

DON'T BE FOOLED BY THE NAME OF THE PRODUCT

Brand-name food companies make products like "Guacamole Dip" that contain no avocado! Instead, they're made with hydrogenated soybean oil and artificial green coloring chemicals. But uninformed consumers keep on buying these products, thinking they're getting avocado dip when, in reality, they're buying green-colored, yummy-tasting dietary poison.

Food names can include words that describe ingredients not found in the food at all. A "cheese" cracker, for example, doesn't have to contain any cheese. A "fruit" product need not contain even a single molecule of fruit. The names are designed to sell products, not to accurately describe the ingredients.

Don't be fooled into thinking that **brown** products are healthier than **white** products. Brown sugar is just white sugar sprayed with a small amount of molasses. Brown eggs aren't any different than white eggs, except that their shells appear brown. Brown bread may not be healthier than white bread either, unless it is made with whole grains.

INGREDIENTS LISTS THAT DON'T INCLUDE CONTAMINANTS

There is no requirement for food ingredient lists to include the names of chemical contaminants, heavy metals, bisphenol-A, PCBs, perchlorate or other toxic substances found in the food. As a result, ingredient lists don't really list what is actually in our food, they only list **what the manufacturer wants you to *believe* is in our food**. In the beginning, food corporations didn't want to be required to list any ingredients at all. They claimed the ingredients were "proprietary knowledge" and that listing them would destroy their business by disclosing their secret manufacturing recipes. In reality, **food companies primarily want to keep consumers ignorant of what is in their products.** That is why there is still no requirement to list various chemical contaminants, pesticides, solvents, acrylamides, PFOA, perchlorate (rocket fuel) and other toxic chemicals that have no nutritional value and may be poisoning our bodies. Nor do they have to list the risks or the substantial impact on the health of consumers. If the ingredient list contains long, chemical-sounding words that you can't pronounce, avoid that item. Remember that **ingredient lists do not have to list chemical contaminants.** The best way to minimize your ingestion of toxic chemicals is to buy organic products, or go with fresh, minimally processed foods.

The ingredients listed on the label aren't the only things in the food. Cancer-causing chemicals, such as acrylamides, may be formed in the food during high-heat processing, yet there is no requirement to list them on the label. Residues of solvents, pesticides and other chemicals may also be present, but also do not have to be listed. The National Uniformity for Food Act, debated in the U.S. Congress, would make it illegal (yes, illegal) for states to require cancer warnings on foods that contain cancer-causing chemicals (http://www.newstarget.com/cancer-causingchemicals.html) [such as California's Proposition 65].

See LivingAnointed.com or do a Google search on articles on the *Food Uniformity Act*

MANIPULATING SERVING SIZES

Food companies have also figured out how to manipulate the serving size of foods in order to make it appear that their products are devoid of harmful ingredients like trans fatty acids. The FDA said any food containing 0.5 grams or less of trans fatty acid per serving is allowed to claim ZERO trans fats on the label. That is FDA logic for you, where 0.5 = 0. But fuzzy math isn't the only game played by the FDA to protect the commercial interests of the industry it claims to regulate.

Exploiting this 0.5 gram loophole, companies arbitrarily reduce the serving sizes of their foods to ridiculous levels, just enough to bring the trans fats down to 0.5 grams per serving. Then they loudly proclaim on the front of the box, "ZERO Trans Fats!" when in reality, the product may be loaded with trans fats.

On the "servings per container" line in the Nutrition Facts box, you may find some high number there that has nothing to do with a realistic portion size. A cookie manufacturer, for example, might claim that **one cookie is an entire "serving" of cookies**. If one cookie contains 0.5 grams of trans fatty acids, the manufacturer can claim the entire package of cookies is "Trans Fat FREE". The package might contain 30 cookies, each with 0.5 grams of trans fats, which comes out to **15 grams** total in the package.

DON'T BE FOOLED BY FALSE STATISTICS

Don't be fooled by fancy sounding herbs or other ingredients that appear very far down the list. There are always two sides to a story. Some food manufacturers that include "goji berries" (real name is Lycium Barbarim) towards the end of the list may be attempting a marketing ploy on the label, giving an illusion of a healthy product. The actual amount of goji berries is miniscule. The nutritional properties are not the same as other Lycium Barbarim. Now as a side note, Young Living Wolfberries (Lycium Barbarim) are the highest nutrient food with unbelievable health and healing properties. Compare the labels for yourself and you will see.

ADHD in children is caused primarily by the consumption of processed food ingredients such as artificial colors and MSG, and refined carbohydrates. 80% of children diagnosed with ADHD who are taken off of processed foods, red dye, and sugars are cured of ADHD in two weeks. (http://www.newstarget.com/artificialcolors.html)

Humans need fat, protein, and carbohydrates to properly perform all their bodily functions. Our brain is 80% fat, we need it to grow and develop. Any diet which eliminates an entire food group for an extended period of time is not sound. This alone is jeopardizing your health. Many food labels say carb-free, fat-free, protein-free, lactose-free, sugar-free, calorie-free, gluten-free, soy-free, and nut-free. When they remove all of those foods, with what are they being replaced? Often they are replaced with chemicals and non-food additives.

Most milk produced in the United States comes from cows injected with synthetic hormones that have been banned in every other advanced nation in the world. These hormones help explain why young girls develop breasts and begin puberty at such a young age and why hormone-related cancers like prostate cancer are being discovered in unprecedented numbers. In order to protect Monsanto, the manufacturer of hormones used in the industry, the USDA currently bans organic milk producers from claiming their milk comes from cows that are not treated with synthetic hormones. Even organic milk is now under fire as the Organic Consumers Association proclaims Horizon milk products are falsely labeled as organic.

The chemical sweetener aspartame, when exposed to warm temperatures for only a few hours, begins to break down into chemicals like formaldehyde and formic acid. Formaldehyde is a potent nerve toxin and causes damage to the eyes, brain, and entire nervous system. Aspartame has been strongly linked to migraines, seizures, blurred vision and many other nervous system problems.

Do you think your produce or vitamin supplements are providing all the vitamins and minerals that you need? Even people who consistently eat good quality fresh fruits and vegetables are not meeting the body's nutritional needs. Our soil is depleted of proper nutrients such as sulfur and minerals. Our produce is grown so fast with the aid of chemicals and **plant breeding** that we are no longer getting whole foods from the ground as our grandparents did.

Not all vitamins and mineral supplements are created equal, nor are they all capable of being absorbed completely into our bloodstream. Many diseases are rooted in vitamin or mineral deficiencies. When your body does not have enough nutrients, it will tap into necessary stores in the body's organs. When this happens long enough, it results in disease.

Now, the presence of genetically modified foods is also increasing. While American consumers remain oblivious, these foods have been introduced into the US food supply without safety testing or even labeling. Already 70% of our U.S. food supply contains **genetically modified,** ingredient including corn, soy, cotton seed oil and canola oil. The following countries have banned **genetically modified food:** Algeria, Egypt, Sri Lanka, Thailand, China, Japan, Philippines, The European Union, Norway, Austria, Germany, United Kingdom, Spain, Italy, Greece, France, Luxembourg, Portugal, Brazil, Paraguay, Saudi Arabia, American Samoa, Cook Islands, Fiji, Kiribati, Federated States of Micronesia, Marshall Islands, Nauru, Papua New Guinea, Samoa, Solomon Islands, Tonga, Tuvalu, Vanuatu, Australia and New Zealand.

This all started from a company called Monsanto, AKA Satan! That may sound harsh to some, but if you do your own investigation into Monsanto, you will see that they are responsible for many problems we have today including **genetically modified food** and aspartame artificial sweeteners. Please watch the movie "Future of Food" or read the book "Seeds of Deception." My website has referrals to this information.

http://www.seedsofdeception.com/Public/Newsletter/index.cfm
http://www.thecampaign.org/

See MSG and Aspartame documents for more information
See "Take Complete Control of Your Health"

The Bad & Terrible Sugar

Processed white sugar compromises your health. It is a long-term chemical poison. Just what damage does sugar do to the human body? The list is endless.

1. Sugar is by far the leading cause of dental deterioration, causing cavities in teeth, bleeding gums, periodontal disease due to excessive plaque build-up, weakening of bone structure, and eventual tooth loss.
2. Sugar is the main cause of diabetes, hyperglycemia, and hypoglycemia.
3. Sugar is either a significant or contributory cause of heart disease, arteriosclerosis, mental illness, depression, senility, hypertension, and cancer.
4. Sugar has a harmful effect on the endocrine system and injures the adrenal glands, pancreas, and the liver, causing blood sugar levels to fluctuate in the component glands.

Processed sugar has a number of other damaging effects on the human body:
- Increases overgrowth of *Candida* (yeast organisms)
- Causes chronic fatigue
- Can trigger binge eating in those with bulimia
- Can intensify PMS symptoms
- Causes hyperactivity in about 50% of children
- Increases or intensifies symptoms of anxiety, irritability and panic attacks
- Breaks down into acid in the body causing inflammation and pain
- Makes it difficult to lose weight because of constantly high insulin levels, causing the body to store carbohydrates as fat.

THE BAD

- **High Fructose Corn Syrup - (HFCS)** - High fructose corn syrup is made by treating corn (which is usually genetically modified corn) with a variety of enzymes, some of which are also genetically modified, to first extract the sugar glucose and then convert some of it into fructose, since fructose tastes sweeter than glucose. The end result is a mixture of 55% fructose and 45% glucose that is called "high fructose corn syrup." Improvements in production occurred in the 1980's making it cheaper than most other sweeteners. A 12-ounce soda can contain 13, or more, teaspoons of sugar in the form of high fructose corn syrup.

- **The dangerous combination: fructose and glucose.** When HFCS breaks down in the intestine, we find near equal amounts of glucose and fructose entering the bloodstream. Fructose short-circuits the glycolytic pathway for glucose. This leads to all the problems associated with sucrose. In addition, HFCS seems to be generating a few of its own problems, epidemic obesity being one of them. Fructose does not stimulate insulin production and also fails to increase "leptin" production, a hormone produced by the body's fat cells. Both of these act to turn off the appetite and control body weight. Also, fructose does not suppress ghrelin, a hormone that works to increase hunger. Peter Havel at UC Davis is doing this interesting work.

Some of the problems associated with high fructose corn syrup are:
- Increased LDL's leading to increased risk of heart disease
- Altered Magnesium balance leading to increased osteoporosis
- Increased risk of Adult Onset Diabetes Mellitus
- Fructose has no enzymes or vitamins thus robbing the body of precious micronutrients
- Fructose interacts with birth control pills and can elevate insulin levels in women on the pill
- Accelerated aging.
- **Brown Sugar** - Sugar crystals sprayed in a molasses syrup, with natural flavor and color; 94% sucrose.
- **Corn syrup** - Made from genetically modified corn and cornstarch. Mostly glucose.
- **Heat-Treated Honey** - When honey is heated (for pasteurization), many of the natural enzymes are destroyed; resulting in a deteriorated quality of honey (reduced freshness, increased level of hydroxymethylfurfural, and reduced enzyme activity). Some bee keepers set out trays of sugar water and or HFCS to feed the bees.
- **Powdered or confectioner's sugar** - pulverized sugar. Often cornstarch is added to prevent caking.
- **Sugar (granulated)** - Refined cane or beet sugar; 100% sucrose. Too much sugar can lead to an unresponsive immune system, diabetes - which will lead to heart disease - renal disease, peripheral vascular disease, diabetic retinitis (blindness), and diabetic peripheral neuropathy (if it's white, it's not right!).

All The "ose's"
- **Dextrose AKA Glucose** - Commonly known as corn sugar and grape sugar. Glucose is the human body's primary source of energy. Most of the carbohydrates you eat are converted to glucose in the body.
- **Fructose** - Found in fruits and honey. The sweetest form of natural sugar. If it is consumed from raw fruit it is acceptable, but when added in a refined form, it is no longer beneficial. Fructose inhibits copper metabolism leading to a deficiency of copper, which can cause increased bone fiagility, anemia, ischemic heart disease, and defective connective tissue formation among others.

- **Galactose** - Sugar found linked to glucose to form lactose, or milk sugar.
- **Lactose** - Sugar found in milk and milk products that is made of glucose and galactose.
- **Maltose** - Called malt sugar. Used in the fermentation of alcohol (beer) by converting starch to sugar.
- **Sucrose** - Common name: **table sugar**

THE TERRIBLE

- **Acesulfame-K** - (ace-K) Introduced in 1967. It is 200 times sweeter than table sugar (sucrose). According to studies, this sweetener is not absorbed in the body but passes through unchanged. This chemical has been reported to break down to acetoacetamide, which has been shown to affect the thyroid in rats, rabbits, and dogs.
- **Aspartame** - Also known as Nutrasweet™, Equal™, Spoonful™, was introduced in 1965. It is a low-calorie sweetener that is 200 times sweeter than sucrose. It is made from two amino acids: L-phenylalanine and L-aspartic acid. The health risks vary and there is a PKU (phenylketonuria) warning on any product that contains Aspartame. Because children lack a "barrier" of protection that prevents the wrong nutrients from entering the brain, doctors have recently suggested that aspartame should not be given to them. It actually can make you gain weight and interferes with some prescription drugs.
- **Saccharin** - It is the oldest artificial sweetener produced in 1878 by a chemist working on coal tar derivatives. The U.S. Congress placed a moratorium on the ban in 1977, now requiring that all saccharin-containing foods display a warning label indicating that saccharin may be a carcinogen (increased potential of cancer, especially bladder cancer). December 14, 2010 the EPA has officially removed saccharin from their list of hazardous commercial chemical products. The EPA stated that "saccharin is no longer considered a potential hazard to human health" Does that mean that it was? It is still on my top terrible sugar list.
- **Sucralose** - Also known as **(Splenda™).** It is a non-caloric sweetener made from sugar and chlorine. It is 600 times sweeter than sugar. Consumption of sucralose can cause side effects such as neurological disorders and stress on the thymus, an organ that is important to the immune system.
- **Truvia** - Truvia is not stevia, it's not natural, but rather made by a mysterious, patented refining process to extract rebiana from the stevia leaf. It contains other ingredients including erythritol and "natural flavors" (whatever they are).

http://www.everydiet.org/articles/sugar_and_alternatives.htm
www.glycemicindex.com   www.DiabeticDigest.com   www.orgs.jmu.edu
http://ezinearticles.com/?The-Dangers-of-High-Fructose-Corn-Syrup&id=28535

What's Wrong With My Cooking Oil?

According to research compiled by Mike Adams in his book entitled ***Poison in the Food: Hydrogenated Oils***, the World Health Organization and hundreds of doctors, researchers and scientists have been warning us for decades about the detrimental health effects of hydrogenated oils. In fact, "hydrogenated oils cause a cell-by-cell failure of the human body by destroying the porosity and flexibility of healthy cell membranes, because they interfere with normal biochemical processes."[1] Margarine, shortening and vegetable oils are fat substances that have been chemically altered. They are known to increase cholesterol, decrease beneficial high-density lipoprotein (HDL), interfere with our liver's detoxification system, and our essential fatty acid function. Dr. Willett at Harvard has shown that "they cause a 53% increase in coronary heart disease." The American Heart Association issued a health warning to avoid food containing these oils.

Consider this list of detrimental health effects caused by hydrogenated oils

- Directly promotes heart disease
- Promotes cancers: breast, prostate, and colon cancer
- Raises LDL and lowers HDL cholesterol
- Raises blood sugar levels and promotes weight gain
- Impairs brain function and damages brain cells
- Accelerates the progress of type 2 diabetes by 39%
- Promotes attention deficit hyperactivity disorder (ADHD)
- Impairs development of the brains of fetuses
- Causes creation of free radicals that promote inflammation
- Weakens cell walls and compromises cellular structure
- Blocks the creation of natural pain-reducing hormones
- Lowers essential fatty acids in the breast milk of nursing mothers
- Impairs immune system function
- Causes dandruff and acne
- Accelerates tumor growth
- Clogs artery walls and promotes atherosclerosis
- Causes gum disease and rotted teeth
- Lowers tissue oxygen intake
- Causes infertility
- Promotes cystic fibrosis
- Directly damages blood vessels
- Causes high blood pressure
- Causes gallbladder disease
- Causes liver disease
- Clogs blood; by making blood cells stick together

First, let's find out the meaning of common words associated with oils. Cholesterol: A soft substance found among the fats in the bloodstream and the body cells. Cholesterol is essential for the body's functioning, and there are two basic types:

1. **Low-Density Lipoproteins (LDL)** carry cholesterol from the liver to the rest of the body. Too much LDL cholesterol in the blood can be deposited on the artery walls.
2. **High-Density Lipoproteins (HDL)** carry cholesterol from the blood back to the liver, which processes the cholesterol for elimination from the body. HDL makes it less likely that excess cholesterol in the blood will be deposited in the arteries.

Also, remember that vegetable oil does not contain cholesterol but helps to promote the formation of it in the body. Cholesterol is only found in foods from animal sources such as poultry, shellfish, eggs, dairy products, lard, and butter.

- **Monounsaturated Fatty Acid (MUFA)** - Monounsaturated fatty acids have one double bond in the form of two carbon atoms double-bonded to each other and, therefore, lack two hydrogen atoms. Your body makes monounsaturated fatty acids from saturated fatty acids and uses them in a number of ways.
- **Polyunsaturated Fatty Acid (PUFA)** - Polyunsaturated fatty acids have two or more pairs of double bonds and, therefore, lack four or more hydrogen atoms. The two polyunsaturated fatty acids found most frequently in our foods are double unsaturated linoleic acid, with two double bonds-also called omega-6; and triple unsaturated linolenic acid, with three double bonds-also called omega-3.
  - Polyunsaturated fats are the absolute WORST oils to use when cooking because these omega-6-rich oils are highly susceptible to heat damage.
  - This category includes common vegetable oils such as:
    Corn   Soy   Safflower   Sunflower   Canola   Peanut
- **Saturated Fats** - A fatty acid is saturated when all available carbon bonds are occupied by a hydrogen atom. They are highly stable, because all the carbon-atom linkages are filled-or saturated-with hydrogen. This means that they do not normally go rancid, even when heated for cooking purposes. They are straight in form and hence pack together easily, so that they form a solid or semisolid fat at room temperature. Your body makes saturated fatty acids from carbohydrates and they are found in animal fats and tropical oils.
- **Refined Oil** - This type of oil has been purified with chemicals to remove any suspended particles, toxic substances, flavor components, color and odor, thereby leaving behind clear and bland oil.
- **Filtered Oil** - Obtained by the traditional cold pressing method, this is filtered once or twice to remove suspended particles.

www.truthpublishing.com/poisonfood p/yprint-cat21284.htm
www.truthpublishing.com/poisonfood - Mercola.com

Yummy Soda Pop

Lets talk about the taboo subject of soda consumption. I get so much grief when I bring up soda. Speaking from experience, I drank soda for 32 years. I know what I am talking about and how overwhelming it is to stop consuming it. It is much easier than you think.

Make a commitment to stop drinking soda for period of time and see how much better you feel. Everything we do is about making better choices. It is possible that you will experience detoxing immediately, so if you get a headache or migraine it will only last 1-3 days. After that you will be fine! Use peppermint to help aleviate the headache.

If you must drink soda, drink regular. Although, I'm not endorsing drinking soda in any way, it is a better choice than drinking diet soda. Drinking soda (diet or regular sugar) is one of the most long-term damaging things that one can do.

15 Negative Effects From Drinking Soda

Soda is useless; it has no nutritional value. It may cause weight gain & obesity, diabetes, weakened bones, osteoporosis, dental carities and erosion, kidney damage, increased blood pressure, metabolic syndrome risk factor, harmful effects on liver, impaired digestive system, dehydration. Most contain high levels of caffeine content and unnatural toxins.

There is so much deception. Please don't succumb to unnecessary health issue for yourself or your children because of soda pop. Peter Piper, a professor of molecular biology and biotechnology at Sheffield University, found that the preservative, Sodium Benzoate, seriously damages living cells. "These chemicals have the ability to cause severe damage to DNA to the point that they totally inactivate it: they knock it out altogether,"

What Happens To Your Body Within An Hour Of Drinking A Soda

In The First 10 minutes: 10 teaspoons of sugar hit your system. (100% of your recommended daily intake.) You don't immediately vomit from the overwhelming sweetness because phosphoric acid cuts the flavor allowing you to keep it down.

- **20 minutes:** Your blood sugar spikes, causing an insulin burst. Your liver responds to this by turning the sugar into fat.
- **40 minutes:** Caffeine absorption is complete. Your pupils dilate, your blood pressure rises, as a response your livers dumps more sugar into your bloodstream. The adenosine receptors in your brain are now blocked, preventing drowsiness.
- **45 minutes:** Your body increases your dopamine production stimulating the pleasure centers of your brain. This is physically the same way heroin works, by the way.

- **60 minutes:** The phosphoric acid binds calcium, magnesium and zinc in your lower intestine, providing a further boost in metabolism. This is compounded by high doses of sugar and artificial sweeteners which also increases the urinary excretion of calcium.
- **60 Minutes:** The caffeine's diuretics properties come into play. (It makes you have to pee.) It is now assured that you'll evacuate the bonded calcium, magnesium and zinc that was headed to your bones as well as sodium, electrolytes and water.
- **60 minutes:** As the rave inside of you dies down you'll start to have a sugar crash. You may become irritable and/or sluggish. You've now, literally, pissed away all the water that was in the Coke. But not before infusing it with valuable nutrients your body could have used for things like having the ability to hydrate your system or build strong bones and teeth. Children's Health, Food Science Research October 24, 2007.

Other statistics on the health dangers of soft drinks include:
- One soda per day increases your risk of diabetes by 85 percent.
- Soda drinkers have higher cancer risk. While the Federal Government has set limits for benzene in drinking water at 5 parts per billion (ppb), researchers have found benzene levels as high as 79 ppb in some soft drinks, and of the 100 brands tested, most had at least some detectable level of benzene present.
- Soda has been shown to cause DNA damage courtesy of sodium benzoate, a common preservative found in many soft drinks, which has the ability to switch off vital parts of your DNA. This could eventually lead to diseases such as cirrhosis of the liver and Parkinson's Disease.
- The average American drinks more than 60 gallons of soft drinks each year.
- One can of soda has about 10 teaspoons of sugar, 150 calories, 30 to 55 mg of caffeine, and is loaded with artificial colors and sulphites. Not to mention the fact that it's also the largest source of dangerous high-fructose modified corn syrup. Mercola.com.

As of April, 2011 the National Corn Growers Association sent this request to the FDA. "We are calling upon the FDA to eliminate the confusion of the safety of high fructose corn syrup," NCGA President Bart Schott said. "Permitting use of the term 'corn sugar' on labels will allow manufactures to more clearly describe high fructose corn syrup as a natural ingredient, nutritionally equivalent to sugar." Unfortunately I'm sure it will be approved soon.

Stick to water, real juice from fresh squeezed fruit, and tea without sweetener. This is just another opportunity to improve your health and well-being.

The reason why we add Young Living oils to the water is because they are for internal use. They bring oxygen to the cells, have the ability to eat the petrochemicals and synthetic substances away from your cells and neurons and they have the ability to change your taste buds very quickly restoring your palate as if you were a baby who has never had soda before. Most think that the desire of taste comes from your taste buds in your mouth. It is not your lips that say "Hey, I want a soda", it is your brain asking for it because it has a memory of how it made you feel when you drank it the last time because of the natural and chemical stimulants in it. When you breath in the oils they go in through the olfactory system right into the Central Nervous System and start working on cleaning off the receptor sites in your nerves system. Even when you drink the oils they still have the ability to affect the limbic section of the brain, (the emotional center) which helps to override the desire to drink the soda because it is cleaning off your receptor sites in the brain and your taste buds in your mouth.

Within 3 weeks I can assure you that you will never want soda again just by drinking Peppermint and Lemon Young Living Essential Oil. If you add 4-6 oz NingXia Red a day to that mix it will take less time. You can give up soda, I did after 32 years!

Hot Dogs & Nitrites

What's wrong with hot dogs? Nitrite additives in hot dogs form carcinogens. The public should petition to ban nitrites! Three different studies have come out in the past year, finding that the consumption of hot dogs can be a risk factor for childhood cancer (preventcancer.com/consumers/food/hotdogs). The study found that children eating more than 12 hot dogs per month have nine times the normal risk of developing childhood leukemia. Children born to mothers who consumed hot dogs one or more times per week during pregnancy have approximately double the risk of developing brain tumors.

How could hot dogs cause cancer? Hot dogs contain nitrites, which are used as preservatives, primarily to combat botulism. During the cooking process, nitrites combine with amines naturally present in meat to form carcinogenic N-nitroso compounds. It is also suspected that nitrites can combine with amines in the human stomach to form N-nitroso compounds. These compounds are known carcinogens and have been associated with cancer of the oral cavity, urinary bladder, esophagus, stomach and brain. Nitrites interact with meat amines to form carcinogenic nitrosamines, which are a major risk factor for childhood cancers.

Unlabeled Toxic Ingredients in Hotdogs and Processed Meats
- Benzene Hexachloride: Carcinogenic
- Dachthal: Carcinogenic (can be contaminated with dioxin); irritant; strong sensitizer
- Dieldrin & DDT: Carcinogenic; xenoestrogen
- Heptachlor: Carcinogenic; neurotoxin; reproductive toxin; xenoestrogen
- Hexachlorobenzene: Carcinogenic; neurotoxic; teratogenic
- Lindane: Carcinogenic; neurotoxic; damage to blood forming cells
- Hormones: Carcinogenic and feminizing
- Antibiotics: Some are carcinogenic, cause allergies and drug resistance

WHAT YOU CAN DO
1. **Buy nitrite free hot dogs and meats.** It's better to err on the side of caution when it comes to our health. There are a few delicious nitrite-free hot dogs on the market. Applegate Farms, *Coleman, Wellshire and Hans* are a few brands. Nitrite-free hot dogs are more perishable than traditional dogs and may be a different color.
2. **Request that your supermarket and schools have nitrite-free hot dogs available.**
3. **Write the FDA and express your concern** that nitrite hot dogs are not labeled for their cancer risk to children. You can mention Cancer Prevention Coalition's petition on hot dogs, docket #: 95P 0112/CP1.

Why French Fries Don't Mold
The Toxic Effects It Has on Your Body
By Austin Kimbrell

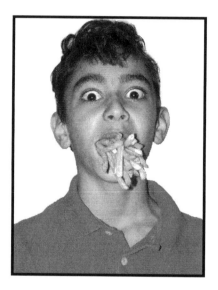

My son Austin (at age 9) decided to do an experiment for the Science Fair at school. His conclusion shocked many. Out of 20 different fast food, sit-down restaurants and frozen french fries only 2 of them molded. That is scary because, if you cut a potato in half it will mold in 2 days. Food is supposed to mold*... If it is real food! Please read Austin's full french fry report at LivingAnointed.com for additional explanation and photos. * (Real food molds under normal conditions, except for foods that naturally dehydrate such as beets, apples, broccoli and gourds). Stacey

As a child, I was french fries biggest fan. It was my favorite for lunch, dinner and snacks. Then when I was 7 years old my mom said lets watch the movie *Super Size Me*. I was confused when I saw the movie because I learned that the french fries I love were not good for me, as I had thought. Then, when I watched Sponge Bob, I saw the grease bubbling as they were cooking the fries and I felt disgusted. But I still wanted them.

Then we did a experiment at home with McDonalds Fries on August 1, 2007, and we saw for ourselves that the fries never molded. Most of the ingredients names I couldn't read. Like Disodium Dihydrogen Pyrophosphate, Sodium Acid Pyrophosphate, Dimethylpolysiloxane, Tertiary butylhydroquinone (TBHQ). I also wanted to know what mold looks like.

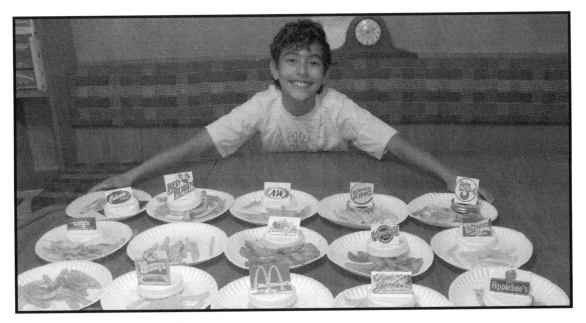

The French Fries That Molded are....

The winner is Red Robin & Fuddruckers! Red Robin and Fuddruckers french fries molded which means they don't have all of the preservatives in them. The hydrogenated and partially hydrogenated oils are not the best, but it is better than the other chemicals and it means it is still a potato! *Caution: Red Robin does have Autolyzed and Hydrolyzed products in their seasoning salt, which is another name for MSG (very toxic), so we don't eat there.

The French Fries That Never Molded Since Nov. 29 2008 to August 12, 2011

A&W	**Famous Dave's**	**RubyTuesday's**
Applebee's	**Gina Restaurant**	**Sonic**
Burger King	**McDonalds's**	**Wendy's**
Culver's	**Olive Garden**	

That means they are laden with chemicals that change the make-up of the food, depriving you of any nutritional value when you eat them and actually harming your body. Do your own experiment and see what fries mold in your area.

Contrary to beliefs it is not because of the oil that they are fried in or the MSG, there is a chemical called Tertiary butylhydroquinone (TBHQ) that prevents food from changing its appearance. Please continue to seek the truth in what is really in our foods.

I miss fries but not as much any more. We eat them once in a while, but only if its Fudruckers. "I don't eat them anymore because they are bad for you, your heart, blood and cholesterol, they have unhealthy chemicals in them that damage you health. They make you gain weight and create liver and gall stones." —Austin Perris Kimbrell

What's In Your Milk?

rBGH (recombinant Bovine Growth Hormone) is a genetically engineered, potent variant of the natural growth hormone produced by cows. Manufactured by Monsanto and supported by the FDA, rBGH milk is claimed to be indistinguishable from natural milk and that it is safe for consumers. It is sold to dairy farmers under the name Posilac. Injection of this hormone forces cows to increase their milk production by about 10%.

- rBGH makes cows sick. Monsanto has been forced to admit to about 20 toxic effects, including mastitis (mastitis is when the breast is inflamed with swelling, redness, tenderness, pain, and infection).
- rBGH milk is contaminated by pus from mastitis, which is treated with antibiotics.
- rBGH milk is chemically and nutritionally different than natural milk; it is super-charged with high levels of a natural growth factor (IGF-1) and rBGH, which is readily absorbed through the gut.
- Excess levels of IGF-1 have been identified as a possible cause of breast, colon, and prostate cancers.IGF-1 blocks natural defense mechanisms that work against early submicroscopic cancers.
- The effect on humans of rGBH is that it contains increased levels of insulin-like growth factor (IGF-1), which is identical in both the cow and human milk, and may be biologically active in humans. Insulin lowers blood sugar levels in humans, and increases cell proliferation. Evidence supports the idea that IGF-1 from rBGH-treated cows may promote cancer of the breast and of the colon in humans who drink such milk.

UNLABELED TOXIC INGREDIENTS IN WHOLE MILK

DDT: Carcinogenic; xenoestrogen.
Dieldrin: Carcinogenic; xenoestrogen.
Heptachlor: Carcinogenic; neurotoxic; reproductive toxin; xenoestrogen.
Hexachlorobenzene: Carcinogenic; neurotoxic; reproductive toxin.
Antibiotics: Some are carcinogenic, cause allergies and drug resistance.

The FDA has sided with Monsanto in opposing labeling of milk produced by drug-treated cows and has gone one step further, opposing labeling of products that are free of rBGH. The FDA has even threatened legal action against milk suppliers and grocers who label their milk as free of the rBGH drug. The FDA says there is "no significant difference" between milk from rBGH-treated cows and milk from cows not treated, and thus a label saying "rBGH-free" would imply a difference that did not exist, and this would constitute false labeling. This more than justifies the rejection of any assurances of its safety. Both the U.S. General Accounting Office (GAO) and the Consumer's Union, publisher of *Consumer Reports* magazine, have warned of the potential hazards to human health caused by consuming products derived from rBGH-treated cows. The sale of Posilac is illegal in virtually every developed country with the exception of the United States.

What about the cows? rBGH will cause suffering to millions of animals, because it is highly addictive for cows. It "revs" their system and forces them to produce a lot more milk, but it also makes them sick. Even the FDA admits that cows injected with rBGH could suffer from increased udder infections (mastitis), severe reproductive problems, digestive disorders, foot and leg ailments, and persistent sores and lacerations.

Every sip of cow's milk contains fifty-nine different bioactive hormones. Milk has always been a hormonal delivery system to humans. It has been found that rBGH contains increased levels of insulin, which, in the diet of young children, can contribute to early signs of puberty. As an effect on humans, antibiotics in milk may increase the danger of low bacterial resistances, cause allergic reactions, and harm the intestinal flora of the person who consumed contaminated milk.

The dairy industry claims that antibiotic residues in the milk couldn't possibly reach the consumer because each tanker of milk is tested and would have to be thrown out if antibiotic residues were found. They explain that every time a milk truck makes a pickup, the farmer's milk is tested. A farmer guilty of providing contaminated milk would then be required to dispose of the milk instead of loading it, therefore it would not be economical.

Only four out of eighty-two commercially used antibiotics are commonly tested. In addition to the fact that so few of these are tested for other antibiotics that are not legal for use end up in our milk. In a May 1992 *Consumers Reports* study, the Center for Science in the Public Interest found 38% of the milk to be adulterated with illegal antibiotics.

LIVING CONDITIONS

If I were to ask you to picture a cow, you would most likely see in your mind a cow grazing in an open pasture enjoying life. That's a lucky organic raised/grass fed cow compared to most of the cows bred for conventional dairy production in this country. The majority of commercial dairy cows don't have the luxury of grazing on open fields. Instead they are kept in intense confinement, in individual stalls, on hard cement floors, hooked up to milking machines and are forced to produce milk nine months out of the year in overcrowded conditions. This is how the average commercial dairy cow spends her short, miserable life of forty-two months on average, compared to twelve to fifteen years for a cow on pasture.

LivingAnointed.com Milk section • sciencenews.org/articles/20031101/food.asp • ejnet.org/bgh/nogood. html • babycenter.com/ • http://www.unsafescience.com/bgh3.html • livinganointed.com http://www.westonaprice.org/transition/dairy.html - look for the photo that shows a cow with large tumors.

What Is Soy?

Are you familiar with soy? There is increasing research on the negative health effects of soy products and soybeans. Cancer, heart disease, sterilization, osteoporosis, brain atrophy, endocrine system disorders, thyroid disease, infertility and blood clotting. Soybeans are high in phytic acid, present in the bran or hulls of all seeds. It's a substance that can block the uptake of essential minerals - calcium, magnesium, copper, iron and especially zinc - in the intestinal tract. Soy also has a high aluminum contamination.

Soybeans are one of the "biotech food" crops that have been genetically modified (GM). In 1995 Monsanto introduced Roundup Ready (RR) soybeans that have been genetically modified to be resistant to the herbicide Roundup that adults, children, infants, fetuses and animal are consuming. The phytoestrogens in soy are potent hormonal influences and can profoundly adversely affect the health of infants up to adults. If you are using soy products please make sure it is organic fermented soy. If not I would not personally feed it to my family.

Were you aware that soy was in all of the following products?

Soy enhanced food products:

Food flavor enhancers (MSG and natural flavors) and emulsifiers, margarine, shortening, salad dressings, cereal, cheese, chips, coffee, creamer, energy bars, flour, grits, ice cream, meat alternatives (burgers, hotdogs, sausage, bacon), miso, pasta, soy protein powder, roasted soy nuts, soy milk, soy nut butter, smoothies, soy sauce (teriyaki, tamari, shoyu), tempeh, Tofu, vegetable oil, olive oil (non cold pressed), whipped topping, yogurt; and most of soybean harvested in the USA are actually used to feed livestock, such as chickens, turkeys, pigs, cows, and fish.

Soy enhanced non-food products:

Candles, caulk, cleaning products, cosmetics, fertilizer, crayons, glycerin, paints, soaps, linoleum, rubber substitutes, plastics, and printing ink, dish washing liquid, fire logs, biodiesel (alternative fuel), furniture, furniture polish, lip balm, skin care, massage oil, oils for machinery, guns, engines and more, pond liners, building insulation, printing inks, soaps and shampoos, socks, stain remover, wood sealer, yarn.

Please visit _LivingAnointed.com_ for more info.

MSG The Excitotoxin

There's a great deal of deception in the labeling of food products found at your local grocery store and even at many health food stores. A disturbing trend I've noticed is that many vegetarian products and grocery items billed as "healthy" or "natural" are using chemical additive taste enhancers found in an ingredient list right on the label. The taste enhancer is MSG - monosodium glutamate - a chemical that has been associated with reproductive disorders, migraine headaches, permanent damage to the endocrine system leading to obesity and other serious disorders.

MSG is a chemical compound that simply does not belong in the body in the concentrations provided by these foods. Food manufacturers use it as a taste enhancer - something to cover up the bland tastes of these foods and make them more appealing to consumers.

MSG is a sodium salt of Glutamic Acid, an amino acid, and a drug. It acts as an excitatory neurotransmitter. It basically causes the nerve cells to discharge an electrical impulse, over-stimulating them and causing them to die. Food companies learned that MSG could increase the flavor and aroma and enhance acceptability of their products. This is why companies in general have no intention of giving up MSG as an additive in their products.

MSG is known to cause uncomfortable reactions for many people. Known reactions include: headaches, heart palpations, intense cravings for the same foods, migraines, hives, mouth eruptions, numbness, tingling, aggressive or agitated behavior, gastrointestinal and reproductive issues, asthma, runny nose, insomnia, seizures, mood swings, panic attacks, diarrhea, cardiac irregularities, addiction, alcoholism, allergy, A.L.S., ADD/ADHD, alzheimer's disease, autism, diabetes, depression, dizziness, epilepsy, fibromyalgia, heat stroke, high blood pressure, hypothyroidism, hypoglycemia, IBS, inflammation, obesity, pituitary tumors, rage/panic disorder, rosacea, sleep disorders, tinnitus, and vision problems. Persons with MS (multiple sclerosis), bronchlospasm (difficulty breathing) in intolerant people with asthma. Other similar auto-immune diseases have been experienced by people very sensitive to MSG. see Dr. Blaylock's book, *Excitotoxins, The Taste That Kills*

Additives that always contain MSG:

- Autolyzed (anything)
- Autolyzed Calcium Caseinate
- Gelatin
- Glutamate
- Glutamic Acid
- Hexametaphosphate Hydrolyzed (anything)
- Monopotassium Glutamate
- Monosodium Glutamate
- Natrium Glutamate
- Plant Protein Extract
- Sodium Caseinate
- Textured Protein
- Yeast Extract
- Yeast Food
- Yeast Nutrient
- Umami

Additives that often contain MSG or create MSG during processing:

- Anything enzyme modified
- Anything fermented
- Anything protein fortified
- Barley malt
- Bouillon and Broth
- Carrageenan
- Enzymes anything
- Seasonings (the word "seasonings")
- Flavor, Flavoring

- Flavors(s) & Flavoring(s)
- Malt extract
- Malt flavoring
- Maltodextrin
- Natural beef flavoring
- Natural beef or chicken
- Natural chicken flavoring
- Natural flavor(s) and flavoring(s)
- Natural pork flavoring
- Pectin Soy protein

- Protease enzymes
- Soy protein concentrate
- Soy protein isolate
- Soy sauce extract
- Spices
- Stock
- Ultra-pasteurized Soy sauce
- Whey protein concentrate
- Whey protein isolate
- Whey protein Protease

MSG is pervasively hidden under other names and aliases so as to go undetected. Most often they appear as "hydrolyzed," "amino acids," and "protein." For example, hydrolyzed proteins appear as pea protein, whey protein, corn protein, etc. If a pea were whole, it would be identified as a pea. Calling an ingredient pea <u>protein</u> indicates that the pea has been hydrolyzed, at least in part, and indicates that processed free glutamic acid (MSG) is present. Relatively new to the list are wheat protein and soy protein. Also, when you see a name for MSG that keeps repeating itself as in "yeast extract, sugar, bluberries, yeast extract, apples...", that is MSG. When you see "whey protein" in a product like chips and yet there is no protein in the serving size, that is another example of MSG.

The presence of MSG has also been reported in soaps, shampoos, hair conditioners, and cosmetics. Low and no-fat milk products, drinks, candy, and chewing gum, binders and fillers for medications, nutrients, supplements (both prescription and non-prescription), enteral feeding materials, and some fluids administered intravenously in hospitals may contain MSG.

Since its introduction into the American food supply fifty years ago, MSG has been added in larger and larger doses to the prepackaged meals, soups, snacks and fast foods we eat everyday. MSG adds flavor to dead, lifeless packaged food. Even food in health food stores can contain MSG. The FDA has set no limits on how much of it can be added to food and the USA national consumption of MSG went from one million pounds in 1950 to 300 times that amount today. Remember by FDA definition, all MSG is "naturally occurring." "Natural" doesn't mean "safe." "Natural" only means that the ingredient started out in nature. However, the "natural flavors" label can be very misleading and the source of much pain, because it can contain anywhere from 12% to 33% MSG - or no MSG at all. The only way to truly know whether MSG is present, and in what amounts, is to write or call the manufacturer.

Under current FDA regulations, when MSG is added to a food, it must be identified as monosodium glutamate in the label's ingredient list. If, however, MSG is part of a spice mix that is purchased from another company, the manufacturer does not have to list the ingredients of that spice mix and may use the words "flavorings or spices". Therefore, under current FDA regulations, even food that uses the *"No MSG"* label may therefore have MSG that is added from a spice mix from another company under current FDA regulations.

The FDA has classified the processed free glutamic acid (MSG) as a constituent food ingredient. According to the FDA, processed free glutamic acid (MSG) is not a food ingredient. There is no requirement that MSG in processed food be listed on product labels. In 1994, the FDA received a citizen's petition requesting changes in labeling requirements for foods that contain MSG. The petition asks for mandatory listing of MSG as an ingredient and the amounts of free glutamic acid on labels of manufactured and processed foods along with a warning that MSG may be harmful to certain groups of people. FDA has not yet taken action on the petition.

Certain **food companies,** described in the *Wall Street Journal* article, are experimenting on how to put more MSG in "MSG-free" foods. Since they will NOT have a label that will alert you to the presence of free glutamic acid, we recommend you avoid ANY and all products that have **blatant misleading advertising.**

Personal story: in my family, MSG has been our biggest problem. It doesn't matter how much we ingest of this neurotoxin, it sizzles off our neurons and destroys us. When Austin was little, he would get very negative and whiny, and then start to cry. When we would ask why he was crying he would always say, "You don't know what's in my head, you don't know what is in my mind". Steve and I would wonder if he had psychiatric issues! Well, we now know it is because of MSG and all of its names. When we started to change our diet, we consumed nothing prepackaged. One day we had a can of Campbell's soup, and everything went down hill. Steve had a migraine, I became a witch with claws and fangs, August retreated, and Austin became negative with whining and complaining. After yelling at the kids, Steve asked me what my problem was and I asked him what his problem was! Austin started crying, so I snapped, "Why are you crying?" He cringed, " You don't know what's in my head, you don't know what is in my mind". Steve said "WHAT DID YOU MAKE FOR DINNER?" It was honestly one of the best and worst moments in our life, because we finally found out what the problem in our home was: MSG!

Dr. Blaylock's book, *Excitotoxins, The Taste That Kills*
Dr. Don Colbert , *Eat This And Live*

http://www.truthinlabeling.com/ • http://www.cnn.com/HEALTH/diet.fitness/9907/23/msg.avoiding/
http://www.fda.gov/opacom/backgrounders/msg.html • http://www.msgtruth.org/avoid.htm
http://freefrommsg.com/ • http://www.naturalnews.com/ • http://www.naturalnews.com/001528.html
*See http://livinganointed.com/links.html for more info.

Effects of Aspartame

In 1981, a revolutionary artificial sweetener was approved for use in dry goods and on tabletops. In 1983, it found its way into carbonated beverages to replace sugar. This notorious additive accounts for more than 75% of all the adverse reactions from food additives that are reported to the FDA.

Aspartame is the technical name for the artificial sweetener used in NutraSweet™951, Ajinomoto™, Equal™ and many other brands. Aspartame is used in many low calorie foods such as yogurts, diet beverages, cereals, vitamins, pharmaceuticals, and chewing gum. This supposedly "healthy alternative" to sugar is widely considered one of the most toxic food additives on the market. It is in diet drinks, many that says "sugar free," "low calorie," "diet," Kool-Aid™, yogurt, cookies, milk, Crystal Light™, children's medications and the list goes on.

What makes Aspartame so dangerous? It is made up of three components: 50% is phenylalanine, 40% is aspartic acid, and 10% is methanol, or wood alcohol. Phenylalanine and aspartic acid are both amino acids. Amino acids are naturally found in the food we eat, specifically in the proteins. They are the building blocks for our bodies, and help us build tissue and muscles. But in nature, amino acids are not ingested singularly. Many types of amino acids are joined together to form protein chains, and that is what we ingest when we sit down to eat. In Aspartame, phenylalanine and aspartic acid are the only amino acids being introduced to the body. There is no protein chain, just single amino acids. It has been found that aspartic acid (when not bound into a protein chain) enters the central nervous system in high concentration and causes the neurons to begin firing rapidly. Fortunately, if you stop ingesting isolated aspartic acid, the damage will also cease.

High levels of isolated phenylalanine can be quite dangerous as well. Research has found that excessive levels of this isolated amino acid causes a decrease in the amount of serotonin in our brains. Decreased serotonin often leads to depression and other mental disorders. When phenylalanine is exposed to warm temperatures, or is stored for a long time, it breaks down into diketopiperazine (DKP), which is a known carcinogen. It is also important to note that in pregnant women phenylalanine easily crosses the placental barrier, and in children under one, also crosses the blood-brain barrier. Infants exposed to high levels of phenylalanine during the pregnancy and later through their mother's milk have an increased risk of birth defects and irreversible brain damage. The brain is unable to protect itself in early stages of childhood or when debilitated by certain chronic conditions. That is why the use of aspartame in presweetened yogurts and vitamins are a huge risk to infants whose parents could be inadvertently damaging their children with only the best intentions in mind.

The third component of Aspartame is methanol. Methanol is commonly known as wood alcohol: a colorless liquid, both poisonous and flammable. Long-term exposure to methanol causes blindness and death. Early symptoms of methanol poisoning include headaches, ear buzzing, dizziness, nausea, gastrointestinal problems, chills, memory lapses, and numbness in the extremities. One particularly alarming aspect of methanol is that at cold temperatures it creates formaldehyde. Formaldehyde, a deadly neurotoxin, is used as an embalming fluid, a disinfectant, a photographic chemical and a leather tanner. Formaldehyde is also a known carcinogen and causes retinal damage, interferes with DNA replication, causes birth defects, and gradually damages the nervous and immune systems. The EPA considers methanol a "cumulative poison," and recommends a limit of no more than 7.8 mg. per day. To put this in perspective, one liter of diet soda contains 56 mg. of methanol, over seven times the EPA limit. By combining several diet sodas, a couple of packages of Aspartame in your morning coffee, and consuming "diet" food during the day, most consumers are exposed to considerably more methanol than the 7.8 mg per day limit.

For 16 years, the FDA denied approval of Aspartame because of compelling evidence that it contributed to brain tumors and other serious disabilities. In 1976, a second task force was created. This time it found the G.D. Searle Co. guilty of faulty and fraudulent product testing, and of knowingly misrepresenting product testing and findings. Donald Rumsfeld (previous Secretary of Defense) left President Ford's administration as Chief of Staff to become the CEO of Aspartame producer G.D. Searle Co. in 1981. Shortly after Rumsfeld became the CEO, and the day after President Reagan took office, Aspartame was quickly approved by FDA Commissioner Arthur Hayes over the objections of the FDA's Public Board of Inquiry. At that time, three FDA scientists came forward to oppose the approval based on their in-house studies of the additive. Hayes ignored these reports and Aspartame was approved. Shortly after Aspartame's approval by the FDA, Hayes joined NutraSweet's public relations firm under a ten year contract at $1,000 a day. Three FDA Commissioners and nine other officers took jobs in the Aspartame industry shortly after it was approved in 1982.

The Food and Drug Administration once listed 92 adverse reactions from 10,000 consumer complaints regarding aspartame and sent the list to all inquirers. In 1996, the FDA stopped accepting complaints and now denies existence of the reports.

www.wnho.net/92_aspartame_symptoms.pdf

ASPARTAME SIDE EFFECTS

Aspartame can travel throughout the body and deposit within any tissue. There are 92 different health side effects associated with Aspartame consumption.

- **Eyes** - Blindness in one or both eyes, decreased vision, blurring, bright flashes, squiggly lines, tunnel vision, decreased night vision, pain in eyes, decreased tears.
- **Ears** - Tinnitus (ringing or buzzing sound), severe intolerance of noise.

- **Neuralgic** - Epileptic seizures, slurring of speech, tremors, headaches, migraines, dizziness, unsteadiness, confusion, memory loss, drowsiness and sleepiness, numbness of the limbs, muscle spasms, severe hyperactivity and restless legs, atypical facial pain.
- **Skin and Allergies** - Itching without a rash, hives, aggravated respiratory allergies such as asthma.
- **Chest** - Palpitations, tachycardia, and shortness of breath, recent high blood pressure.
- **Gastrointestinal** - Nausea, diarrhea, sometimes with blood in stools, abdominal pain, pain when swallowing.
- **Psychological/Psychiatric** - Severe depression, personality changes, irritability, aggression, anxiety, insomnia, and phobias.
- **Endocrine and Metabolic** - Loss of control of diabetes, menstrual changes, severe PMS, thinning or loss of hair, weight loss, fluid retention, low blood sugar (hypoglycemia).
- **Additional Symptoms of Aspartame** - Frequency of voiding and burning during urination, excessive thirst, fluid retention, leg swelling, bloating, increased susceptibility to infection, birth defects (including mental retardation), suicidal tendencies, irreversible brain damage, peptic ulcers, increased craving for sweets, hyperactivity in children, severe depression, aggressive behavior or death.

Aspartame may trigger, mimic, or cause the following illnesses:

- ALS
- Alzheimer's Disease
- Attention Deficit Disorder (ADD)
- Brain tumors
- Chronic Fatigue Syndrome
- Diabetes
- MS
- Epilepsy
- Epstein-Barr
- Fibromyalgia
- Grave's Disease
- Hypothyroidism
- Lupus
- Lyme Disease
- Lymphoma
- Mercury fillings sensitivity
- Meniere's Disease
- Multiple Sclerosis
- Non-Hodgkin's
- Parkinson's disease
- Post-Polio Syndrome
- Vertigo

www.wnho.net/the_ecologist_aspartame_report.htm • www.drtrudipratt.com/library_aspartame.html
www.ehso.com/ehshome/aspartame.php
www.totse.com/en/politics/green_planet/additivetheswe171840.html

See "Take Complete Control of Your Health", and "NeuroToxin"

The Dark Side of Mold

Many things have been taught when in comes to getting rid of mold. Most of the common remedies don't really work. We do know that exposure to mold happens more often than we think. It can happen everyday! The negative long-term health effects may start with a cough or sore throat. The effects become much greater over time.

I was blessed to be able to interview Dr. Close, Author of Nature's Mold Rx. The following information was drawn from this interview and moldrx4u.com. Dr. Close has answered many common questions. He explains why YLEO's Thieves blend may be the best solution. The Thieves oil not only kills mold but also digests it. This has been proven.

How People Are Exposed to Mold

Mold exposure can produce and mimic disease in several ways. The most common is inhalation. Other forms of exposure are through skin contact, ingestion and open orifice such as the mouth, eyes, and ears. Mold allergy by inhalation of mold spores through the respiratory tract and the sensitization through the GI tract may be an alternate pathogenic route. With this in mind we realize that exposure can allow mold to grow inside our bodies. Mold can grow in our sinus cavities, lungs and intestines. This may provoke hypersensitivity reactions." FDA Science Forum 2004. www.accessdata.fda.gov/Science-Forums/forum04/K-16.htm

Common Health Effects Associated with Exposure to Mold Toxins (Mycotoxins)

Some symptoms common with mold exposure that may be mistaken for other ailments are asthma, hypersensitivity, pneumonia, allergies, sneezing, wheezing, cough, irritation of the nose, mouth, or throat, nasal stuffiness and runny nose, and red, itchy or watery eyes, shortness of breath, cough, muscle aches, chills, fever, night sweats, weight loss, profound fatigue, mucous membrane irritation, skin rash, nausea, immune system suppression, acute or chronic liver damage, acute or chronic central nervous system damage, endocrine effects, and cancer. http://www.cdc.gov/mold/stachy.htm

"Approximately 100,000 species of fungi exists; fewer than 500 fungal species have been described as human pathogens that can cause infections." CDC http://www.cdc.gov/mmwr/preview/mmwrhtml/rr5508a1.htm

Facts About Top 5 Mythological Treatments

The most common myth about killing mold is that harsh chemicals are perfect for doing the job. Another mistake we make is that other common treatments are safe and effective. The fact is that bleach, ozone generators, and UV lights are ineffective and can be dangerous.

1. **Bleach** is Ineffective – And May Be Hazardous To Your Health.
   - Bleach is ineffective and not recommended for use on porous surfaces such as concrete, wood, wallpaper, sheet rock, grout, books, or clothing.
   - Cleaning stirs up mold spores and releases them into the air, creating more mold related health problems and allergic reactions.
   - Bleach only treats the surface. It does not kill or eliminate airborne mold spores.
   - Bleach is 3-6% Sodium Hypochlorite and 94% to 97% water. The Sodium Hypochlorite evaporates, leaving water behind to foster the growth of mold.
   - Bleach is successful in bleaching out the color of the surviving mold, leaving it undetectable to the necked eye.
   - Mold usually returns in less than 24 hours after using bleach.
2. **Ozone generators** may pose multiple hazards to your health. Using the ozone generator at a sufficient level to kill the mold may cause the mold to oxidize. "This results in the production of off-gasses of harmful contaminants that have adverse effects in the air you breath." Air purifiers producing ozone are banned by California, citing studies that it leads to lung damage. Also, ozone machines will not address the source of the mold. www.epa.gov/ttncaaa1/t1/fr_notices/o3naaqs.pdf and www.epa.gov/osp/bosc/pdf/pm0508rpt.pdf
3. **UV** only kills mold in the air that is exposed directly to the UV light.
   - UV does not treat surfaces. It only treats air streams that are directly exposed to the UV.
   - UV has no impact on the source of mold in buildings.
4. **Tear It Out, Remove It, Replace It, Tear It Down**
   - Repairing leaks is essential to eliminating mold problems, however, this option can be very costly and does not remove mold spores from the air.
5. **Chlorine dioxide and other fumigants**
   - Not practical for occupied buildings, harmful to humans, pets.
   - Chlorine dioxide will damage metals fasteners, nails, and electrical wiring.
   - Mold will rebound using these poisonous agents. www.moldrx4u.com and †http://www.azdhs.gov/phs/oeh/invsurv/air_qual/pdf/moldfact.pdf

Did You Know

1. Mold affects pets as well as people with the same side effects and diseases.
2. Most people are not aware of the serious health effects of mold.
3. You can get mold out of carpet but generally not carpet padding.
4. Spores are easily released into the air when molded material is dried.
5. If you have mold in your home it can appear to only affect one person.
6. Air/heating ducts and ventilation systems do get contaminated with mold spores.
7. Once mold becomes airborne, it may spread/travel to other areas to germinate and colonize. It travels through air vents, out windows and into neighbors' windows, on toys, clothes etc. Certain types of mold can float or be carried (clothes, fur, etc.) up to a distance of 100 feet.
8. It is mandatory to properly seal or contain the room or area that has been exposed to mold while you are performing the clean up process. "Keep air circulation confined to the area." Use plastic sheeting sealed with duct tape to cover doorways, vents, and other openings of occupied areas of the home or building.

The Solution to Mold

The results of hundreds of case studies, verified by an independent EPA-approved environmental laboratory, have shown that organically produced concentrated plant extracts (also known as essential oils), such as the blend Thieves will digest the mold. When Thieves oils are diffused in the air, they eliminate mold spores in the air and on surfaces in as little as 24 hours.

1. Thieves Oil Blend -15 ml - amount need depends on square footage of space. "Thieves will go anywhere there is air movement."
2. Thieves Household Cleaner.
3. "Use PPE Personal Protection Equipment, which includes: a mask, earplugs, goggles with no holes, gloves, and body suit, per Dr. Close."
4. An Essential Oil Cold-Air Diffuser with a 6.0 watts pump. "This Diffuser will work for up to 1000 square feet of space with 8-10 foot ceilings, depending on mold infestation level, size and layout of the rooms. The mold diffuser can be purchased through Stacey Kimbrell at 810.423.5721 or Dr. Close's website MoldRx4U.com.

I suggest you purchase the book "Nature's Mold RX" authored by Dr. Edward Close, PhD, PE and the DVD "Toxic Mold" to understand everything in more detail.

Microwave Ovens Destroy Our Food's Nutritional Value

The rise of widespread nutritional deficiencies in the western world correlates almost perfectly with the introduction of the microwave oven. This is no coincidence. Microwave ovens heat food through a process of creating molecular friction, but this same molecular friction quickly destroys the delicate molecules of vitamins and phytonutrients (plant medicines) naturally found in foods. Research compiled by Lita Lee, PhD (www.litalee.com) shows that microwaving foods decreases the foods value by up to 60-90% (vitamins and other plant-based nutrients that prevent disease, boost immune function and enhance health).

Eating raw broccoli provides you with natural anti-cancer medicine that's extremely effective at halting the growth of cancer tumors. But microwaving that broccoli destroys the anti-cancer nutrients, rendering the food "dead" and nutritionally depleted. There is even some evidence to suggest that microwaving destroys the natural harmony in water molecules, creating an energetic pattern of chaos in the water found in all foods microwaved. In fact, the common term of "nuking" your food is coincidentally appropriate: using a microwave is a bit like dropping a nuclear bomb on your food, diminishing the nutritional value.

WHY MICROWAVE USERS ARE SO UNHEALTHY

Humans are the only animals on the planet who destroy the nutritional value of their food before eating it. All other animals consume food in its natural, unprocessed state. The invention of the microwave and its mass adoption by the population coincides with the onset of obesity in developed nations around the world. Not only did the microwave make it convenient to eat more obesity-promoting foods, it also destroys much of the nutritional content of those foods, leaving consumers overfed and malnourished. In other words, **people eat too many calories but not enough real nutrition.** The result is, of course, what we see today: epidemic rates of diabetes, cancer, heart disease, depression, kidney failure, liver disorders and much more. These diseases are all caused by a combination of malnutrition, exposure to toxic chemicals, lack of exercise, etc.

Microwaving is, technically, a form of food irradiation. I find it interesting that people who say they would never eat "irradiated" food have no hesitation about microwaving their food. In fact, microwaves were originally called "radar ranges." When microwaves were first introduced in the 1970's, they were proudly advertised as radar ranges. Do yourself a favor: **toss your microwave.** It is much easier to avoid using the microwave if you don't have one around. It will clear up counter space, save you electricity and greatly enhance your dietary habits. When you need to heat something, heat it in a toaster oven, Vita Mix or the stove top. Better yet, strive to eat more of a raw, unprocessed diet, where the best nutritional value can be found.

Toxic Plastic Bottles and Containers

Many products contain toxic chemicals that may have detrimental health impacts for children exposed during critical stages of development. In this report (see below for link), we analyze the extent to which five popular brands of baby bottles leach bisphenol A (BPA), a developmental, neural, and reproductive toxicant, into liquids coming into contact with them. The U.S. Centers for Disease Control and Prevention (USCDCP) found bisphenol A in the urine of over 95% of people they tested. Alarmingly, the median level of bisphenol A in humans is higher than the level that causes adverse effects in animal studies. www.cdc.gov/exposurereport/executive_summary.html.

Bisphenol A is a developmental, neural, and reproductive toxicant - Scientists have linked very low doses of bisphenol A exposure to cancers, impaired immune function, early puberty, obesity, diabetes, and hyperactivity, among other problems. In addition, *ABC News* reported on 4/15/08 that bisphenol A was found in the urine of adults and children, umbilical cords, placentas, and is suspected to cause breast cancer and prostate cancer later in life.

Exposure to Bisphenol A is widespread - Bisphenol A is most commonly used to make clear polycarbonate plastic for consumer products, such as baby bottles and water bottles. This is also used as a liner in canned foods. Through use, this plastic breaks down and leaches bisphenol A into liquids and foods with which they come into contact.

AVOID THE FOLLOWING

Popular baby bottles leach bisphenol A at harmful levels. The bottles tested from all five brands leached bisphenol A at levels found to cause harm in numerous laboratory studies, including:

- Avent
- Dr. Brown's
- Evenflo
- Gerber
- Playtex

Please reference the links at the end of this chapter for the most updated information on baby bottles.

You should avoid buying and using #3, #6, and #7 Plastics

#3 Polyvinyl Chlorides or Vinyl (V, PC or PVC)
- Used in some cling wraps, some "soft" bottles.
- PVC is hazardous in all of its phases: manufacturing, the products themselves in the home, and in the disposal of it.
- One of the most toxic plastics, PVC is often used to make food packaging and in the production of plumbing and construction materials. PVC is commonly used in teethers and soft squeeze toys for young children, beach balls, bath toys, and dolls.

- To soften PVC into these flexible forms, various toxic chemicals are added as "plasticizers." Traces of these chemicals, known as adipates and phthalates, can leak out of PVC into your food. Some phthalates have been linked to cancer, kidney and liver damage, harm to developing reproductive organs, and premature breast development in baby girls. Inhaling these chemicals can also worsen asthma in children.

#6 Polystyrene (PS)
- Used in foam "clam-shell"-type containers, meat and bakery trays, and in its rigid form, clear take-out containers, and some plastic cutlery and cups.
- #6 plastic may leach styrene into the food it touches. A recent study in Environmental Health Perspectives, an online journal, concluded that some styrene compounds leaching from food containers are estrogenic (meaning they can disrupt normal hormonal functioning). ehp03.niehs.nih.gov.
- Styrene is also classified as a possible human carcinogen by the World Health Organization's International Agency.

#7 (Other)
- Usually Polycarbonate on the underside, used in 5-gallon water bottles, some baby bottles, and some metal can linings.
- #7 can release its primary building block, bisphenol A, which is another suspected hormone disruptor, into liquids and foods.

RECOMMENDATIONS

You can take a few simple actions to limit exposure to these and other toxic chemicals. <u>Use Glass or stainless steel</u> when possible. Choose plastic food containers, bottles and cups made using:

1. **#1** polyethylene terephthalate (PET or PETE) used for most clear beverage bottles.
2. **#2** high-density polyethylene (HDPE) used for "cloudy" milk and water jugs, opaque food bottles.
3. **#4** low-density polyethylene (LDPE) used in food storage bags and some bottles.
4. **#5** polypropylene (PP) used in rigid containers, including some baby bottles, and some cups and bowls. **Adiri, Nurture Pure, Think Baby, Medela, Born Free and First Years** are better choices.

What can I do to reduce my exposure to the chemicals in plastic?

1. Avoid canned foods, including baby formula, which may contain bisphenol A in their lining.
2. Avoid foods wrapped in plastic. Choose butcher paper, waxed paper or cellulose bags.
3. Do not microwave food in plastic or polystyrene.
4. Do not put plastics in the dishwasher, and dispose of any plastic containers or dishware that look scratched or hazy.

5. Choose #1 (PETE) or #2 (HDPE) whenever plastic cannot be avoided!
6. Choose packaging that is made from truly recyclable materials: paper, glass and metal.
7. Do not let children put plastic toys in their mouths. Parents should visit LivingAnointed.com/protect-our-babies.html.
8. Choose wooden toys or toys labeled "PVC-free". Most children's products are not labeled.
9. Buy in bulk, whenever possible. It is the least-packaged option.
10. Bring cloth bags to your supermarket to carry groceries home.
11. Call manufacturers to find out whether products contain bisphenol A or phthalates.

Should I be concerned about using plastic in the microwave?

The Center for Environmental Oncology of UPCI contends that NO plastics (including Styrofoam, wraps or containers) should be used in the microwave. (See previous chapter "Microwave Ovens Destroy Our Food's Nutritional Value").

Contact your local government and policymakers

Visit "http://www.usa.gov/contact/elected.shtml" to contact your State Governor, Congress Representative, Senator and other officials. Stand up for your rights to be informed in order to protect your children and family.

- **Phase Out Hazardous Chemicals** - Based on the weight of the scientific evidence showing the harm caused by exposure to bisphenol A, the government should act now.
- **Inform Consumers about the Presence of Dangerous Chemicals** - Parents currently have little information to guide their decisions when purchasing products for their family. Manufacturers should be required to label children's products with the name of any potentially dangerous chemicals and the specific health risks associated with the chemicals.
- **Reform Chemicals Policy** - Chemical manufacturers should be required to provide all potential hazards and health-effects information to the government so agencies can begin to assess the thousands of chemicals currently on the market. Next, pre-market hazard and health-effects testing should be required. Finally, the California Environmental Protection Agency must have the authority to protect public health by banning or restricting the use of a chemical if evidence shows that it can harm human health.

http://www.checnet.org/healthehouse/education/articles-detail.asp?Main_ID=24
To learn about the alternatives to PVC that are available.
http://www.environmentcalifornia.org

Top 25 Harmful or Carcinogenic Ingredients in Our Home

Are you aware that most of the personal care products used today contain cancer-causing agents? How about your everyday cleaners? Are they safe? Here is a list of the top 25 unwanted ingredients commonly found in your home and their side effects. See Document (Toxic Chemicals List) for more information.

1. **Isopropyl Alcohol** - This is a solvent and denaturant (poisonous substance that changes another substance's natural qualities). Isopropyl alcohol is found in hair, body and makeup products, after-shave lotions, and fragrances. This petroleum-derived substance is also used in antifreeze and as a solvent in shellac. According to **Consumer Guide of Cosmetic Ingredients,** inhalation or ingestion may cause headaches, flushed skin, dizziness, depression, nausea, vomiting and narcosis.

2. **Mineral Oil** - Baby oil is mineral oil. This substance, a commonly used petroleum ingredient, coats the skin just like plastic wrap covers any given vessel. The skin's natural immune barrier is disrupted as this plastic coating inhibits its ability to breathe and absorb (moisture and nutrition). Your skin's ability to release toxins is impeded by this "plastic wrap," which promotes acne and other disorders. In addition, by slowing down normal cell development, mineral oil causes the skin to age prematurely.

3. **Propylene Glycol (PG) (PEG) (PROPANEDIOL, DIHYDROXYPROPANE, METH-YLETHYLENE GLYCOL, PROPANE)** - As a wetting agent and solvent, this ingredient is actually the active component in antifreeze. There is no difference between the PG used in industry (brake and hydraulic fluid, paint, floor wax) and PG used in personal care products. It is used in industry to break down protein and cellular structure (what the skin is made of) stripping the natural moisture factor, yet it is in make-up, hair products, lotions, after-shave, deodorants, mouthwashes, toothpaste and processed food. The EPA requires workers to wear protective gloves, clothing, and goggles when working with this toxic substance because of its ability to quickly penetrate the skin. Human test have shown skin contact can cause contact dermatitis, kidney damage, and liver abnormalities. It can inhibit cell growth and damage membranes, causing rashes, dry skin and surface damage. NOTE: visit LivingAnointed.com to print an Anti-Freeze container showing the name Propylene Glycol. I actually have the container proving this. It is really hard to find the Low Tox Anti-Freeze containers any more.

4. **Sodium Lauryl Sulfate (SLS) and Sodium Laureth Sulfate (SLES)** - Used as detergents and surfactants, these closely related compounds are found in car wash soaps, garage floor cleaners and engine degreasers. Surprisingly, both are used in cosmetics, toothpaste, hair conditioner and about 90% of all shampoos and products that foam. According to the American College of Toxicology, both SLS/ SLES can cause malformation in children's eyes and damage to the immune system, especially within the skin. Skin layers may separate and inflame due to its protein denaturing properties. It is possibly the most dangerous of all ingredients in personal care products.

5. **Chlorine** - Exposure to chlorine in tap water, showers, swimming pools, laundry products, cleaning agents, food processing, sewage systems and many other venues can affect health by contributing to asthma, hay fever, anemia, bronchitis, circulatory collapse, confusion, delirium, diabetes, dizziness, heart disease, high blood pressure and nausea. Exposure can also lead to irritation of the eyes, mouth, nose, throat, lung, skin, and stomach.

6. **DEA (diethanolamine), MEA (momoethanolamine), and TEA (triethanolamine)** - These chemicals are used in conjunction with the compound being neutralized. One should therefore look for names like Cocamide DEA or MEA, Lauramide DEA, etc. These are hormone-disrupting chemicals and are known to form cancer causing nitrates and nitrosamines. They are commonly found in products that foam including bubble baths, body washes, shampoos, soaps and facial cleansers. *CBS'* Roberta Baskin revealed that a recent government report shows DEA and MEA are readily absorbed through the skin.

7. **Artificial Colors and Dyes** - Some artificial colors, such as Blue 1 and Green 3, are carcinogenic. Impurities found in commercial batches of other cosmetic colors such as D&C Red 33, FD&C Yellow 5, and FD&C Yellow 6 have been shown to cause cancer not only when ingested, but also when applied to the skin. Some artificial coal tar colors contain heavy metal impurities including arsenic and lead, which are carcinogenic. The use of permanent or semi-permanent hair color products, particularly black and dark brown colors, is associated with increased incidence of human cancer, including lymphoma, myeloma, and Hodgkin's disease.

8. **Fragrance** - Fragrance is present in most deodorants, shampoos, sunscreens, skin care and baby products. Many of the compounds in fragrance are carcinogenic or otherwise toxic. "Fragrance" on a label can indicate the presence of up to 4,000 separate ingredients. Most or all of them are synthetic. The FDA reports have included headaches, dizziness, rashes, skin discoloration, coughing, vomiting, and allergic skin irritation as possible side effects. "Exposure to fragrances can affect the central nervous system, causing depression, hyperactivity, irritability, inability to cope, and other behavioral changes," says Dr. R. Blaylock and Dr. G. Young.

9. **Imidazolidinyl Urea and DMDM Hydantoin** - These release formaldehyde into your body. Go to formaldehyde.MSDS to see how it can irritate the respiratory system, cause skin reactions and trigger heart palpitations. Exposure may cause joint pain, allergies, depression, headaches, chest pains, ear infections, chronic fatigue, dizziness and loss of sleep. It can also aggravate coughs and colds and trigger asthma. Serious side effects include weakening of the immune system, carcinogenic, mutagenic for bacteria and/or yeast and mutagenic cells.

10. **Bronopol (2-bromo-2-nitropropane-1, 3-diol)** - Bronopol may break down in products into formaldehyde and also cause the formation of carcinogenic nitrosamines under certain conditions. "Natural" and both expensive and inexpensive lines of cosmetics often use this chemical. Many baby care products may also include bronopol.

11. **1, 2 Dioxane in Surfactants/detergent's** - A wide range of personal products including shampoos, hair conditioners, cleansers, lotions, creams, household soaps and cleaners contain surfactants or detergents such as ethoxylated alcohols, polysorbates, and laureths. These ingredients are generally contaminated with high concentrations of the highly volatile 1,4 dioxane, which is both readily inhaled and absorbed through the skin. 1,4 dioxane has caused cancer in lab animals.

12. **Talcum Powder** - (talc) is carcinogenic. Inhaling talc and using it in the genital area, where its use is associated with increased risk of ovarian and lung cancer, are the primary ways this substance poses a carcinogenic hazard.

13. **Lanolin** - Lanolin itself is perfectly safe. But cosmetic-grade lanolin can be contaminated with carcinogenic pesticides such as DDT, dieldrin, and lindane, in addition to other neurotoxin pesticides.

14. **Parabens (methyl-, ethyl-, propyl-, butyl-, isobutyl-)** - disrupt hormones, a study found that butyl paraben damaged sperm formation in the testes of mice. Parabens break down in the body into p-hydroxybenzoic acid, which has estrogenic activity in human breast-cancer cell cultures.

15. **Silica** - Crystalline silica is carcinogenic.

16. **Air Fresheners** - Most air fresheners work by coating your nasal passages with an oily film, or by releasing a nerve-deadening agent. Known toxins are: formaldehyde, a highly toxic known carcinogen and phenol, which can cause swelling, burning, peeling, and breaking out (if comes in contact with skin) in hives and could cause coma and death.   nrdc.org/media/2007/070919.asp.

17. **Ammonia** - It is a very volatile chemical, damaging the eyes, respiratory tract and skin.

18. **Bleach** - It is a strong corrosive. It irritates or burns the skin, eyes and respiratory tract. It may cause pulmonary edema or vomiting. WARNING: never mix bleach with ammonia it causes DEADLY fumes.

19. **Dishwasher Detergents** - Highly concentrated chlorine. It is the number one cause of child poisonings.

20. **Drain Cleaner** - Drain cleaners contain lye, hydrochloric acid or Trichloroethane. Lye: caustic, burns skin and eyes, if ingested will damage esophagus and stomach. Hydrochloric acid: corrosive, eye and skin irritant, damages kidneys, liver, digestive tract. Trichloroethane: eye, skin irritant, nervous system depressant; damages liver, kidneys.

21. **Furniture Polish** - Petroleum Distillates: highly flammable, can cause skin and lung cancer. Phenol: (see Air fresheners) Nitrobenzene: absorbed through skin, extremely toxic.

22. **Mold and Mildew Cleaners** - Chemicals contained are: Sodium hypochlorite, a corrosive, irritates or burns skin and eyes, causes fluid in the lungs which can lead to coma or death. Formaldehyde: highly toxic, known carcinogen. Irritant to eyes, nose, throat and skin. Causes nausea, headaches, nose-bleeds, dizziness, memory loss and shortness of breath.

23. **Oven Cleaner** - Sodium Hydroxide (Lye): Caustic, strong irritant, causes burns to both skin & eyes. Inhibits reflexes, severe tissue damage if swallowed.

24. **Carpet & Upholstery Shampoo** - These formulas are designed to overpower the stain itself by using highly toxic substances. Perchloretylene: known carcinogen, damages liver, kidney and nervous system. Ammonium Hydroxide: corrosive, extremely irritating to eyes, skin and respiratory tract. Protect kids safety while crawling. It can cause Kawasaki Syndrome.

25. **Toilet Bowl Cleaners** - Hydrochloric acid: highly corrosive, irritant to both skin and eyes, also damages kidneys and liver. Hypochlorite Bleach: corrosive irritates or burns eyes, skin and respiratory tract. May cause pulmonary edema, vomiting, or coma if ingested.

THE EFFECT

Immune Systems Under Attack

Our immune systems face a daily **attack, assault, or ambush** of stresses. In an otherwise healthy person, common signs of a weakened immune system include frequent colds as well as chronic allergies. Allergic reactions occur when the body perceives allergens (such as pollen, dust, or mold) as poisons. It then secretes histamine, creating familiar allergy symptoms. They're not really poisons, but if your immune system is already compromised, your body reacts as if they are. Allergy suffering has greatly increased in the past 30 years, yet the allergens haven't really changed. Trees, grasses, pets, dust, and mold have always been around. But our environment has changed.

You need to watch the movie Rave Diet; this will open your eyes to see how devastating the changes in our food supply, mainly our livestock, are effecting our health. The animals have been increasingly treated with antibiotics, growth hormones, and steroids. They are fed treated feed with fungicides, pesticides, herbicides, genetically modified foods (GMO) as well as other ground-up animals and aquatics.

Today our standard American diet (SAD) is heavily dependent on processed convenience foods full of additives and dyes, and new synthetic foods with hydrogenated or artificial fats and artificial sweeteners. These are all substances that the body doesn't recognize as nourishment, but rather as toxins that have to be eliminated. The immune system is busy dealing with these foreign substances, and may not have the reserves necessary to deal with for the common allergens, germs, and viruses.

80% of your immune system is located in your intestinal tract and the other 20% can be found in your Thymus Gland.

You must keep your digestive system working properly!

A diet of poor quality foods also creates a digestive system that becomes unbalanced, resulting in partially digested proteins being absorbed into the body fluids. This then causes the immune system to overreact, wasting valuable energy that could be used elsewhere in its fight against viruses. A compromised digestive system leads to poor absorption of nutrients. A healthy whole food diet and positive thinking are really the building blocks of a long, healthy, and strong immune system, reducing the risk of disease and allowing your body to naturally heal itself.

The **immune system** is a collection of mechanisms within an *organism* that protects against *disease* by identifying and killing *pathogens* and *tumor* cells. It detects a wide variety of agents, from *viruses* to *parasitic worms,* and needs to distinguish them from the organism's own healthy *cells* and *tissues* in order to function properly. Detection of the immune system being under attack is complicated as pathogens adapt and develop new ways to successfully infect the *host* organism.

To survive this challenge, several mechanisms have evolved that recognize and neutralize pathogens; watch the Osmosis Jones movie. Even simple *unicellular* organisms such as *bacteria* possess *enzyme* systems that protect against viral infections. The human immune system consists of many types of *proteins*, cells, *organs*, and tissues. As part of this more complex immune response, the vertebrate system adapts over time to recognize particular pathogens more efficiently. The adaptation process creates *immunological memories* and allows even more effective protection during future encounters with these pathogens. That is why we need to reprogram our cells, nerves, and DNA so it can create a new memory of a healthy state. Using Young Living Essential Oils can clean off the cells, nerves receptor sites, rid Candida off your intestinal lining, and restore DNA, so that you can improve your immune system functions.

Disorders in the immune system can cause disease. *Immunodeficiency* diseases occur when the immune system is less active than normal, resulting in recurring and life-threatening infections. When one or more of the components of the immune system is inactive, the ability of the immune system to respond to pathogens is diminished. **Chemical saturation and *malnutrition* are the most common causes of immunodeficiency.** Diets lacking sufficient oxygen and whole food nutrition are associated with impaired cellular functions.

Autoimmunity

Overactive immune responses comprise the other end of immune dysfunction, particularly the **auto-immune disorders.** Here, the immune system fails to properly distinguish between self and non-self, and either attacks a part or attacks parts of the body.

Eating Right for a Healthy Immune System

An immune-friendly diet consists of a variety of healthy foods-fruits, vegetables, grains, legumes, nuts, seeds, and protein dense foods. Regular use of sugar, nicotine, alcohol, caffeine, and chemicals often defeats the efforts of your immune system to protect you. Common food allergens that irritate your immune system are distracting it, keeping it off track. The most common food allergens are cow's milk, eggs, wheat, soy, sugar, tomatoes, corn, nuts, particularly peanuts, and yeast. Some common food reactions include headache, nasal congestion, an upset digestive system, fatigue, fast pulse, frequent or dramatic mood changes, water retention, and difficulty losing weight. Check your sensitivity to these foods by eliminating one at a time for about two weeks. See how you feel. Try rotating potential allergenic foods in and out of your diet. Some doctors are willing to conduct testing to determine whether you have food sensitivities or allergies.

"Take Complete Control of Your Health...," *Living Balanced* p. 47

http://health.howstuffworks.com/immune-system1.htm

Immune Booster Tonic

If you are sick now with the cold or flu or just need an immune boost take this tonic twice a day. To build up your immune system take 1/4 cup of this daily when the cold season starts. I suggest using whole organic lemons including the rinds, which are full of nutrients.

Freshly squeezed juice from 4 to 8 lemons (about 2 cups)
>   9 - 12 cloves peeled garlic (1 bulb)
>   1/2 to 3/4 cup of honey or raw blue agave
>   1 onion, peeled and cut into chunks
>   1/2 to 1 tsp cayenne pepper (liquid works better)
>   1 thumb-sized piece fresh peeled ginger (or 1 tsp dried)
>   2 quarts water

1. Put all ingredients, and 1/2 of the water, in blender and blend until smooth. Then add rest of water.
2. If it's too potent to drink, you can boil it for a minute or so.
3. Shake before each use. You can heat it up to have as a hot tea or drink mixture cold.

My mother-in-law, Madeline Marks, gave me this tonic to take 17 years ago. I have used it throughout the years for my own family and friends. Hint: when making this for friends you may not want to tell them what is in it until they have finished it. Thanks Mom!

Inflammation = Degenerative Disease

Contains excerpts from *Nutrition in a Nutshell Book* by Bonnie C. Minsky

Inflammation has long been linked to rheumatoid arthritis, osteoarthritis, chronic inflammation, allergies, asthma, Alzheimer's disease, cancer, diabetes, digestive disorders, heart disease, hormonal imbalances, bladder problems, and osteoporosis. Inflammation causes tissues to become inflamed and results in redness, heat, swelling, pain, and loss of function. When acute inflammation doesn't shut down, it becomes chronic and causes damage to the injured tissues. Inflammatory stimuli, such as bacterial infection, trauma, ischemic events, stress-related events, toxic exposures, allergens, and chronic viral infections activate the inflammatory response. According to the health experts the biggest culprit in causing abnormal inflammation is the "standard American diet" (SAD) of heavily processed convenience and fast foods. Sugar is one of the most serious causes of inflammation, rapid aging, and weight gain. Sugary foods quickly elevate blood sugar, creating an insulin release along with free radicals that oxidize fats. When oxidized, the fats form plaque deposits in our arteries, leading to disease. Therefore a diet high in sweets, pasta, fruit juices, cereals and even rice cakes can actually lead to heart disease. Insulin release also increases stored body fat and the release of pro-inflammatory chemicals causing cell damage and accelerated aging. Inflammation equals aging. Inflammation is the reason you get wrinkles, why you can become forgetful, why you can be irritable and depressed, and why you lose the healthy bloom of youth. Inflammation is what causes arthritic pain, stiffness when using your muscles, the wheezing of asthma, and the discomfort of allergies. It is even possible that the progression of atherosclerosis is directly related to chronic inflammation in up to 50% of cases. Excess **acid** production also increases the inflammatory response leading to the loss of bone and joint tissues.

Ca·tarrh = An inflammatory affection of any mucous membrane, a response of the body tissues to injury or irritation; characterized by pain and swelling and redness and heat.

1. Catarrh of the bladder is called cystitis.
2. Catarrh of the stomach is called gastritis.
3. Catarrh of the large intestine is called colitis.
4. Catarrh of the ear is called otitis.
5. Catarrh of the bronchi is called bronchitis (hay fever, asthma, COPD, etc.)
6. Catarrh of the heart is called carditis, pericarditis, endocarditis, etc.
7. Catarrh of the joints is called arthritis.
8. Catarrh of the veins is called phlebitis.

See "Take Complete Control of Your Health"

How Do You Doo?

Boy… this is a crappy subject! The thing everybody does, but no one really wants to talk about, so "How Do You Doo?"

In 2007 when we first learned about health, I found out it is not normal to go Number 2 every 4-5 days. Imagine my surprise! For as long as I can remember my son and I did just that. The key here is I thought it was NORMAL! Why is this important? Because the intestinal tract is 80% of the immune system and if it is not cleaned out and working correctly your body will never function properly! No mater what age you are, get your bowels working 3 times a day. Holy BM Bat Man, is that possible. Why yes it is Robin. My kids hated it when I first brought out the poop calendar. "Ah mom, that's gross." And… I don't care what they say to you, get out your new poo, (aka: bowel movements, stools, dump, crap, elimination) calendar and find how often, what it looks like and how it smells. Document this for 2-4 weeks. Then start the cleansing process.

How the bowel works

From the moment food enters your mouth, and the chewing process begins you are producing enymes. As the food goes down, hydrochloric acid, and digestive enzymes, bile, and other secretions all work to give each meal the consistency of split pea soup. While your digestive cells are absorbing the nutrients from what you have eaten; sugars, starches, fats, vitamins, minerals, and other nutrients, waste products continue traveling down through the intestine.

The remaining waste "our feces", consists of water, indigestible fiber, and undigested food. When the feces enter the colon they are considered toxic and are expelled from the body. The large bowel/colon absorbs water back into the body and the feces become more solid. When feces reach the rectum, the urge to pass a bowel movement is felt.

What Should an Ideal Bowel Movement Look and Smell Like?

An ideal bowel movement (IBM) is medium brown and should look like type 4 (see page 47). An IBM should happen 3 times a day and be approximately 4 to 8 inches long. IBM should be in one piece, like the shape and size of a banana and tapered at the end. IBM should leave the body easily with no straining or discomfort. There should be little to no gas or odor. IBM should not take more than a minute to completely evacuate.

What do the colors and smells mean?

There are many different reason for fowl or discolored stools; drinks, foods, dyes natural and chemical, medication, alcohol, bacterial overgrowth, infections etc. so take a minute and investigate what you've taken in.

Rancid, Foul - may mean too high an intake of animal proteins or an imbalance of intestinal bacteria. This means you definitely need to perform a colon cleansing.

Mucous Present - may indicate too many unhealthy foods or foods that you are allergic to. Whitish mucus in stool may indicate there is inflammation in the intestines. When doing a colon cleanse you will see mucus come out as well.

Parasites - 70% of parasites are microscopic and are not visible to the human eye. There are up to 3000 different types. If you see something white/tan that is anywhere from the size of a grain of rice to ramen noodles to a pencil in diameter whether its round or flat, that is a parasite. I say some have fangs and claws, do a cleanse just because, most people have them. See cleansing section.

Loose Stool - Abdominal bloating, lack of energy, and poor appetite can be signs of a condition known as spleen deficiency. It doesn't necessarily involve your actual spleen, but it is linked to tiredness and weak digestion brought on by stress and poor diet.

Pencil Thin and Ribbon Like - A polyp or growth in your colon that narrows the passage for stool. This is also known as a spleen deficiency or bowel obstruction. Benign rectal polyps, prostate enlargement, colon or prostate cancer are some of the conditions that can cause obstruction.

Large and Floating with greasy film on the Toilet Water- Malabsorption--your digestive system isn't getting the full nutritional use of food.

Bouts of Diarrhea and Constipation - Irritable bowel syndrome. This chronic condition can be aggravated by red meat, spices, sugar, alcohol, lack of fiber, allergy-causing foods, irregular hours, and chaotic relationships.

Black, Tarry, and Sticky - Internal bleeding in the upper digestive tract, stomach or esophagus. The black color comes from digested blood cells. High amounts of iron, medications, foods dark in color.

Very Dark Brown - You drank red wine last night or have too much salt or not enough vegetables in your diet.

Glowing Red or Megenta - bleeding from hemorrhoids or anal fissures. Red dyes or you've eaten a lot of reddish foods such as beets.

Light Green - You're consuming too much sugar, or too many fruits and vegetables with not enough grains or salt.

Yellow Stool - Can indicate that food is passing through the digestive tract relatively quickly. Also, can result from GERD, insuffient bile output, and be a sign of a bacterial infection in the intestines

Orange – Any food with artificial yellow or orange coloring or aluminum hydroxide (antacids)

Pale or Clay – Colored may indicate a bile duct obstruction, problem with gallbladder or liver. Medications, alcohol, tumor, gallstones, giardia parasitic infection, hepatitis, chronic pancreatitis, or cirrhosis. Also, aluminum hydroxide (antacids).

Blood or Mucus - Hemorrhoids, an overgrowth of certain bacteria in your gastrointestinal tract, colitis (inflammation of the colon), Crohn's disease (also known as inflammatory bowel disease), or colon cancer. Red blood usually means the ailment is located near the end of your digestive tract, whereas black blood signals partially digested blood coming from an ailment higher up the tract. Seek medical advice promptly.

"The Bowl Truth" Patrick Donovan, N.D – www.Mayoclinic.com, www.About.com/health

How Do You Doo Chart

What Should an Ideal Bowel Movement Look and Smell Like?

An ideal bowel movement (IBM) is medium brown and should look like type 4. A IBM should happen 3 times a day and be approximately 4 to 8 inches long. IBM should be in one piece, like the shape and size of a banana and tapered at the end. IBM should leave the body easily with no straining or discomfort. There should be little to no gas or odor. IBM should not take more than a minute to completely evacuate.

The Seven Common Types of Stools Per the Bristol Stool Chart

	Type 1: separate hard lumps, like nuts (hard to pass). Constipation- even if you're defecating frequently. Not enough water. Possible causes are eating too much dry food, including protein, and not enough vegetables and raw foods, laxative abuse, worries, or irritable bowel syndrome.
	Type 2: sausage-shaped but lumpy. This type is also constipation. See type 1 for same causes.
	Type 3: like a sausage but with cracks on its surface = optimal
	Type 4: like a sausage or snake, smooth and soft = Ideal way to pass. This is our goal to achieve, when having a BM.
	Type 5: soft blobs with clear-cut edges, easily passed through digestive system. Soft diarrhea- may indicated a possible risk for bowel disease. You also may be toxic and need an intestinal cleansing.
	Type 6: fluffy pieces with ragged edges, a mushy stool. Diarrhea- indicated you may be toxic and need an intestinal cleansing.
	Type 7: loose, watery, no solid pieces, and sometimes can see undigested foods Diarrhea- possible causes are food, poisoning lactose intolerance, antibiotics, antacids, dietary changes, travel, anxiety, stress, inflammatory bowel disease, or irritable bowel syndrome.

The Bristol Stool Chart was first published in the Scandinavian Journal of Gastroenterology in 1997. This version is a compilation and hand illustrated by the Kimbrell Family with clay. LivingAnointed.com

Healthy Cell 101

Human life begins at conception. When the sperm of the male joins the egg of the female, a single cell forms. This single cell contains DNA, which is a blueprint of what the body will be like, including the sex, eye color, hair, etc. After the sperm and egg unite, that original cell divides into two cells (each with its own DNA) and the two cells become four cells and the four become eight and the eight become 16, etc. These cells divide and multiply at an unbelievable rate of speed for the next 11 months. About 2 months after birth, the body has its full complement of cells, around 100,000,000,000 (one hundred trillion).

Throughout life, <u>every 4 weeks, the entire outer layer of our skin is replaced. Every 2 months, practically every cell in our heart muscle, cartilage and joints is rebuilt.</u> It is even possible to regenerate meniscus tears and deteriorating discs through proper nutrients (docereclinics.com). So, 2 to 3 years from this very moment, every cell in our body will have been replaced with a new cell.

What kind of body will it be? Will this new body be weaker or stronger? The new cell is totally dependent on the building materials we provide it, which are the foods we eat, the liquids we drink, and the air we breathe. Proper cell care is the key to our health, energy, strength, mental stability, and an immune system that will resist illnesses.

1. **Cell 101** - Cells are the fundamental units of life, the bricks from which all your tissues and organs are made. Your cells are constantly communicating with each other, responding to your environment and to the signals they receive from what you touch and how you move. In order for our cells to function properly, they must have a healthy environment. This includes maintaining a body temperature of 98.6 degrees; a proper acid / alkaline balance of about 7.4 pH; and providing the cells with pure air and water, all necessary minerals, and keeping them free from toxic waste and stress. Cells will live, function, and recreate themselves without any problems. Your cells keep your DNA safe from damage, and provide energy for everything you do. These are the two most important factors. Your DNA is stored within your cell in the nucleus, and your cell has many ways to keep it safe; however, research has shown that a poor diet, one low in antioxidants and other important phytonutrients and environmental exposure to toxins, like pesticides, can cause your DNA to become damaged. This damage, called a mutation, can affect the ability of your cells to produce energy, can cause your cells to die early resulting in *compromised tissue or inflammation,* which is the root cause of all illness and disease including cancer.

2. **Cell Food** - Maintaining healthy cells involves a variety of vitamins and minerals as well as other dietary components. Providing nutrients to your cells means eating chemical free whole RAW foods, whole grains, fruits, vegetables and grass feed animal products. Every step in the processing of food takes it further from the way

the body cells need to be nourished. Without this range of nutrients and phytonutrients, the membranes in your cells can become brittle, develop holes (become leaky), are unable to function properly, and unable to protect your cell's DNA and energy-producing machinery. Once the cell is unprotected, your DNA can develop mutations, which can cause the cell to be unable to function or to become malignant (cancerous). Damage to your energy-producing machinery can decrease energy production and lead to an increase in generation of free radicals, causing more damage and destroying your cell's ability to function entirely.

3. **Cell Exercise** - In order to ensure proper functioning of all cells, body fluids need to be kept moving. This can be accomplished only by exercise. Exercise is absolutely essential for building and maintaining healthy cells. Exercise puts oxygen into the blood, keeps the lymphatic fluid moving, and helps maintain the general health of the entire body. It strengthens and nourishes all the various organs and systems of the body. When exercise is neglected, all the cells—muscles, organs, glands, the circulatory and respiratory systems, etc.—become weakened and sluggish, and this, in turn, leads to all manners of physical breakdown.

4. **Cell Protection** - The body's defenses include the skin, mucous membranes, friendly bacteria, tear glands, fever, lymphatic system, fighter cells, and the immune system. The immune system contains about a trillion cells called lymphocytes and about 100 trillion molecules called antibodies. These cells provide protection against all microscopic enemies seeking to enter the body. We immobilize our immune system by putting *harmful* substances into our body! For example, *white table sugar* paralyzes the immune system. Ingesting just 9 teaspoons of sugar (1 soda = 10 tsp.) in a day will immobilize the immune system by about 33%, while approximately 30 tsp. of sugar will wipe out the immune system from even functioning that day. High processed fat intake and white table salt seriously impair the functions of the immune system. *Caffeine* suppresses the immune system by upsetting the delicate mineral balance, which deprives the immune system of essential minerals. All drugs and pain killers adversely affect the immune system, even aspirin.

5. **Positive Mental Attitude** - All through history attitude has been recognized as an important ingredient in *quality of life*. Laughter and enjoyment can release substances in the body which enhance the immune system, while sadness, anger, or worry can actually depress the immune system.

It is so exciting to realize that we can control the health of our body cells by proper diet and exercise!!! Based on what we put into our bodies, we determine what our body will be made of, and how well it will function. Therefore, we can prevent sickness!!! Simply cleansing the body of toxins and providing the cells with the proper nutritional materials can correct almost all sickness and disease.

See "Take Complete Control of Your Health"

Rev. George Malkmus & http://whfoods.org/index.html & Answers.com

http://www.whfoods.com/genpage.php?tname=faq&dbid=19 great visual on cells.

Neurotoxins

This is my new, favorite subject, NEURONS! You're going to learn that neurons are our communication center for our whole body. There are products that we use daily that contain neurotoxic chemicals. We consume them unknowingly via our food, drinks, baby products, perfumes, air-fresheners, candles, skin care, cleaning supplies, yard supplies, etc. They are easily absorbed through the skin, inhaled or ingested. These chemicals are linked to cancer, birth defects, learning disabilities, dementia, Alzheimer's (sometimes), and many other health problems. Most of us use more than one of these adulterated products in a day and small amounts of these toxins can add up significantly enough to do harm.

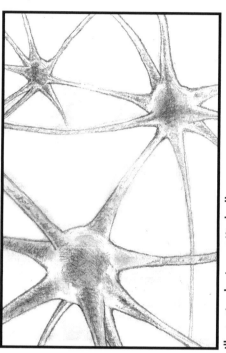

Illustration by August Kimbrell

Consider, if I at 180 lbs. share a bowl of soup full of MSG with Austin at age 9 and 80 lbs, who will receive more of the neurotoxin? If I use a lotion full of chemicals on myself, and my nephew at age two weighing 30 lbs, who will absorb more chemicals? We have to open our eyes!

The next two paragraphs are excerpts from *The Owner's Manual* by Dr. Michael F. Roizen and Dr. Mehmet Oz (pp. 72-73). I want to show you medical doctors are stating this information is true. Also, I encourage you to purchase *Excitotoxins, the Taste that Kills* by Russell L. Blaylock, MD and *Eat this and Live!* by Dr. Don Colbert.

Neurons - You have 100 billion neurons in your brain, which, if stretched out in length, would reach thirty thousand miles. Each of these nerve cells contains pieces of information that need to be transmitted to other neurons so that your body can properly function. Neurons hold the information, but unless it's communicated to other neuron, it's virtually useless. This is where the edges of neurons come into play. They're called dendrites and they're performing like baseball catchers... They receive the pitch sent to them from other neurons. Specifically, the dendrite can influence how the signal is sent, received, and transmitted to other neurons.

Neurotransmitters - These are the chemical messengers in your brain--like baseballs being tossed back and forth. When you turn a neuron on, the neurotransmitters ring or blare out to help send or receive information between neurons. When you experience neurological disorders, the cause often stems from a flaw in the neurotransmitter--if it can't transport one piece of information to another neuron, then you have difficulty completing a specific task. Also, a natural decline in the function of certain neurotransmitters is believed to make you more vulnerable to such conditions as dementia and depression.

Neurotoxins - These cause neurological damage, affect brain development, altered functions and behavioral changes, dizziness, headaches, epileptic-like seizures, itching, nausea, nervous system and reproductive disorders, high blood pressure, and also pass from pregnant mothers to their unborn child.

- Lead, aluminum, mercury, etc. are Neurotoxins that cause brain damage, and are found in vaccinations, food, skin care and much more.
- Aspartame, NutraSweet, Equal, sucralose (Splenda), neotame, saccharin, Sweet 'N Low, Sweet One, acesulfamek, Sunette, Sweet-n-Safe. Breaks down in the body to phenylalanine (a neurotoxin causing seizures), aspartic acid (damages the developing brain) and methanol (turns into formaldehyde).
- Monosodium glutamate, MSG, 622, Autolyzed Plant Protein, Autolyzed Yeast, Calcium Casein-ate, Gelatin, Glutamate, Glutamic Acid, Hydrolyzed Oat Flour, Hydrolyzed Plant Protein (HPP), Hydrolyzed Protein, Hydrolyzed Vegetable Protein (HVP), Monopotassium Glutamate, Natrium Glutamate, Plant Protein Extract, Sodium Caseinate, Textured Protein, Yeast Extract, Yeast Food, or Yeast Nutrient.

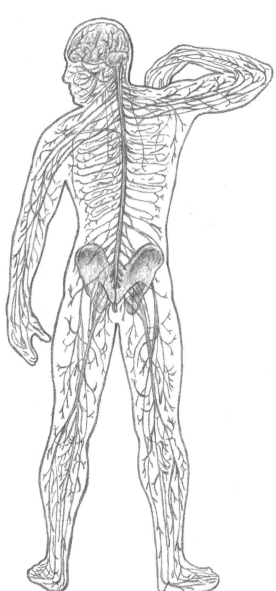

Image courtesy of bodylink.co.nz   re-illustrated by Steve Kimbrell

Cholesterol Myths & Truths

Whether you are a meat eater or vegetarian, please read the myths and truths provided. It is very important to make sure we get the good fats in order for your body to function properly. *This information has been provided and approved by The Weston A. Price Foundation to be included in this book.*

Myths & Truths

MYTH: People with high cholesterol are more prone to heart attacks.

TRUTH: Young and middle-aged men with cholesterol levels over 350 are slightly more at risk for heart attacks. Those who have cholesterol levels just below 350 are at no greater risk than those whose cholesterol is very low. For elderly men and for women of all ages, high cholesterol is associated with a longer lifespan.

MYTH: Cholesterol & saturated fat clog arteries.

TRUTH: There is very little cholesterol or saturated fat in the arterial plaque or clogs. Most of the material is a calcium deposit akin to lime and most of the fatty acids are unsaturated.

MYTH: Eating saturated fat and cholesterol-rich foods will cause cholesterol levels to rise and make people more susceptible to heart disease.

TRUTH: Many studies show no relationship between diet and cholesterol levels; there is no evidence that saturated fat and cholesterol-rich food contribute to heart disease. As Americans have cut back on saturated fat and cholesterol-rich foods, rates of heart disease have gone up.

MYTH: Cholesterol-lowering drugs have saved many lives.

TRUTH: In the two most recent trials, involving over 10,000 subjects, cholesterol-lowering drugs did not result in any improvement in outcome.

MYTH: Countries that have a high consumption of animal fat and cholesterol have higher rates of heart disease.

TRUTH: There are many exceptions to this observation, such as France and Spain. Furthermore, an association (called a "risk factor") is not the same as a cause. In wealthy countries where people eat a lot of animal foods, many other factors exist that can contribute to heart disease.

Dangers of Statin Drugs

Modern cholesterol-lowering drugs act by inhibiting an enzyme (HMG-CoA reductase) needed for the formation of cholesterol in the liver. These HMG-CoA reductase inhibitors, called statins, are sold as Lipitor, Mevacor, Pravacol, Zocor, etc.

Weakness and Muscle Wasting - This is the most common side effect of statin drugs, occurring in as many as one in three users. Muscle aches and pains, back pain, heel pain, weakness and slurring of speech result from statin interference with the production of Coenzyme Q10 (Co-Q10), needed for the muscles to function. These side effects are more common in active people and may not show up until three years after onset of treatment.

Heart Failure - Rates of heart failure have doubled since the advent of statin drugs. The heart is a muscle that depends on a plentiful supply of Co-Q10.

Polyneyneyneuropathy - Tingling and pain in the hands and feet as well as difficulty walking occur frequently in those taking statins, conditions often blamed on "old age" rather than on the drug.

Cognitive Impairment - Many patients have reported memory loss and brain fog, including total global amnesia (episodes of complete memory loss). The implications for pilots and those driving cars and trucks are profound.

Cancer - In every study with rodents to date, statins have caused cancer. Most human trials are not carried out long enough to detect any increase in cancer rates, but in one trial, breast cancer rates of those taking a statin were 1500 percent higher than those of controls.

Depression - Numerous studies have linked low cholesterol with depression.

If It Isn't Cholesterol, What Causes Heart Disease?

Many scientists have put forth valid theories for the epidemic of heart disease in western societies. They include:

Deficiency of Vitamins A and D - Back in the 1930s, Weston A. Price, DDS, observed that rates of heart attack rose during periods of the year when levels of these fat-soluble vitamins in local butter went down.

Deficiencies of Vitamins B6, B12 and FOLIC ACID - Kilmer McCully, MD, PhD, demonstrated that these deficiencies lead to elevated levels of homocysteine, a marker for heart disease.

Trans Fatty Acids - Fred Kummerow, PhD, and many others have linked heart disease to the replacement of saturated fats with trans fatty acids; saturated fats actually protect against heart disease in many ways.

Mineral Deficiencies - Deficiencies of magnesium, copper and vanadium have been linked to heart disease.

Milk Pasteurization - J.C. Annand, a British researcher, observed an increase in heart disease in districts that implemented pasteurization compared to those where milk was still sold unpasteurized.

Stress: Heart attacks often occur after a period of stress, which depletes the body of many nutrients.

Unfortunately, little research money is available for researchers to study these theories; most research on heart disease is funded through the National Heart, Lung, and Blood Institute, which is firmly committed to the flawed hypothesis that cholesterol and saturated fat cause heart disease.

The Many Vital Roles of Cholesterol

- Cholesterol is produced by almost every cell in the body.
- Cholesterol in cell membranes makes cells waterproof so there can be different chemistry on the inside and the outside of the cell.
- Cholesterol is nature's repair substance, used to repair wounds, including tears and irritations in the arteries.
- Many important hormones are made of cholesterol, including hormones that regulate mineral metabolism and blood sugar, hormones that help us deal with stress, and all the sex hormones, such as testosterone, estrogen and progesterone.
- Cholesterol is vital to the function of the brain and nervous system.
- Cholesterol protects us against depression; it plays a role in the utilization of seratonin, the body's "feel-good" chemical.
- The bile salts, needed for the digestion of fats, are made from cholesterol.
- Cholesterol is the precursor of vitamin D, which is formed by the action of ultra-violet (UV-B) light on cholesterol in the skin.
- Cholesterol is a powerful antioxidant that protects us against free radicals and therefore against cancer.
- Cholesterol, especially LDL-cholesterol (the so-called bad cholesterol), helps fight infection.

How to Avoid Heart Disease

- Don't worry about your cholesterol-the stress of unnecessary worry can contribute to heart disease.
- Do not take cholesterol-lowering drugs-they contribute to heart failure.
- Avoid processed food, especially foods containing processed vegetable oils and trans fats.
- Eat the meat, fat and organ meats of grass-fed animals.
- Eat plenty of wild-caught seafood.
- Take cod liver oil and consume plenty of butter from grass-fed cows to ensure adequate levels of vitamins A, D and K.
- Maintain a healthy weight—neither too heavy nor too thin.
- Engage in moderate exercise outdoors.
- High-protein diets lacking the nutrients supplied by grassfed/organice raised animal fats can deplete vitamin A, leading to heart disease.
- Do not smoke.
- Avoid exposure to environmental toxins.

Sources and Further Information

The Cholesterol Myths by Uffe Ravnskov, MD, PhD www.ravnskov.nu/cholesterol.htm www.westonaprice.org/modern-diseases

The Impact of Acidosis On Our Organs

Acidosis is a condition where the pH of the blood serum becomes excessively acidic. This is not to be confused with acid from the stomach. Acidic blood can stress the liver and eventually lead to many forms of chronic and degenerative diseases. Dietary modification is the first course to pursue in raising the pH making it more alkaline. Your pH is really a sign of how your body is managing your mineral reserves. Acidosis will decrease the body's ability to absorb minerals and other nutrients, decrease the energy production in the cells, decrease its ability to repair damaged cells, decrease its ability to detoxify heavy metals, make tumor cells thrive, and make the body more susceptible to fatigue and illness. Try to avoid antibiotics, because they kill the beneficial bacteria in your intestines while also killing the bad bacteria. An acidic pH can occur from an acid-forming diet, emotional stress, toxic overload, and/or immune reactions or any process that deprives the cells of oxygen and other nutrients.

Over-the-counter antacids appear to help because they neutralize these organic acids and the pain diminishes. The antacids aggravate the situation because they have left the stomach more alkaline. Now an even greater amount of hydrochloric acid must be produced to finish digestion. Apple cider vinegar is rich in malic acid, which increases the acidity of digestive fluids causing them to flow faster, which improves digestion. You will need to investigate why you have this condition, but in the meantime take action. You can manually manipulate your pH balance by using 1/2 teaspoon baking soda in 8oz of water, alkaline from Young Living, drinking fresh lemon water, or Braggs Organic Apple Cider Vinegar 1-2 tsps in 8oz of water.

Foods: Are they Acid or Alkaline-forming?

Food's acid or alkaline-forming tendency in the body has nothing to do with the actual pH of the food itself. For example, lemons are alkaline-forming in the body. Although lemons are very acidic, after digestion and assimilation they become very alkaline. Likewise, meat will test alkaline before digestion, but it leaves acidic residue in the body.

It is important that your daily dietary intake of food naturally acts to balance your body's pH. To restore health, the diet should consist of 75% alkaline and 25% acid-forming foods; once healthy 60% alkaline and 40% acid foods.

What is the Impact of Acidosis on Our Organs?

Colon - The colon must be kept clean of accumulated acid wastes. Poisons collect on the colon walls causing diarrhea or constipation and will harden and reabsorb into the bloodstream. Good bowel action (complete elimination) must be done at least 2 times per day. Bowel movements that do not completely clear the body of its daily poisons are also reabsorbed.

Stomach - Digestive difficulties (belching, bloating, sensitivity at the waist, intestinal gas, regurgitation, hiccups, lack or limitation of appetite, nausea, vomiting, diarrhea, constipation, and colic in children) may indicate vagus nerve problems and possible hiatal hernia syndrome, which can produce acid residue throughout the system. Hiatus hernia can quickly reduce necessary hydrochloric acid in the stomach. Without the proper hydrochloric acid breakdown of foods, the foods become too acidic. Many people think that too much acid causes heartburn in the stomach. But heartburn occurs when there is not enough of the right kind of acid to digest food properly. The stomach needs hydrochloric acid to break down food. When there is not enough hydrochloric acid, the food starts to putrefy, producing organic acids, which cause heartburn and indigestion.

Liver - The liver has over 300 functions including processing acid toxins from the blood, producing numerous alkaline enzymes for the system, and it is your first line of defense against any poison. All the nourishment obtained through the gastrointestinal tract enters the blood by way of the liver. The load on the liver is much heavier when acid waste products are constantly floating in the blood. If the liver becomes too congested with protein acid wastes, death is imminent.

Pancreas - The pancreas is highly dependent on a correct alkaline diet. All aspects of pancreatic function reduce excess acidity and regulate blood sugar balance (so you don't get diabetes). To have proper blood sugar balance, you must maintain an alkaline-forming diet.

Small Intestines - The small intestines are crucial to life. They are essential for proper assimilation of food and producing lymphocytes for the lymphatic system's wide-ranging nodal network. They also produce large amounts of the enzyme which is a major alkalizing substance.

Kidneys - In an adult, about 1 liter of blood per minute passes through the kidneys. By executing their primary duty, the kidneys keep the blood alkaline and extract acid. Kidneys that are over-stressed with too much acidity create kidney stones, which are composed of waste acid cells and mineral salts that have become gummed together in a waste acid substance. Therefore, by reducing acid-forming products from entering the body, the chances of avoiding this painful condition are better.

Heart - The heart is one of the most alkaline-dependent organs in the body. It is partly innervated by the vagus nerve, which functions best in an alkaline environment. Acid wastes alter a correct heartbeat. These wastes rob the blood of proper oxygenation and degeneration of the heart follows. An alkaline system creates ideal heart function.

Lymphatic System - There are 600-700 lymph glands in the body. Lymph fluid carries nutrition to the cells and removes acid waste products. Lymph fluid flows best in an alkaline environment. When the body is overly acidic, it slows down, creating one of the most chronic, long-term, life-threatening conditions. Hindered lymph flow increases tissue acid storage. Not drinking enough purified water will also slow the lymph flow. Waste products from foods that are not properly digested are reabsorbed into general circulation via the lymphatic ducts of the small intestine.

How Negative Emotions Create Acidity - Have you ever been so upset with someone or something that you get an upset stomach? All negative emotions create an acidic environment. Have you ever heard anyone say you are letting your problems "eat away at you" or "get the best of you"? Fear is the underlining cause of most diseases. It will undermine your life and your health. Fear causes anger. Anger causes hate. Hate will consume you with continual suffering. Love and understanding cleanse and heal the body creating an alkaline environment within you.

Other Symptoms of Acidosis

Cardiovascular damage, weight gain, obesity and diabetes, bladder conditions, kidney stones, immune deficiency, acceleration of free radical damage, hormonal problems, premature aging, osteoporosis and joint pain, aching muscles and lactic acid buildup, leg cramps and spasms, slow digestion and elimination, yeast/fungal overgrowth, lack of energy, fatigue, loss of drive, joy, enthusiasm, depressive tendencies, increased stress, headaches, inflammation of the corneas, eyelids, loose and painful teeth, inflamed sensitive gums, mouth and stomach ulcers, nails that are thin and split easily.

How to test your own pH Balance

You can purchase pH test strips from a health food store or pharmacy. Tear off two three-inch strips. When awakened, before you brush your teeth, drink, or eat, do a saliva test. Compare the color to a pH color chart that comes with the test strips. Next, measure the pH of your urination mid stream by collecting the urine in a plastic or glass (not paper) cup and dip the test strip. Test yourself four days in a row, and then take the average of those four days. Loging the numbers the same time every day. You want to start with the 2nd urination of the day. You can retest a few weeks after changing your eating habits. *Don't get in a cycle of testing your urine hourly or daily. This just causes unnecessary stress!*

WHAT CAN YOU DO if you have an "Acidic" body?

- **Exercise** - Moderate exercise is alkalizing to the body. Excessive exercise (past the point of exhaustion) can create an acidic problem due to lactic acid buildup. People who are acidic usually feel worse from exercise because their detoxification organs are not working properly, due to excessive acid in the tissues. Yet without exercise, acid and toxin buildup are likely. Because waste disposal is done in liquid form through urination and perspiration, it is imperative that we drink plenty of water. Since all waste products are acidic, the best kind of water is alkaline water.
- **Water** - Drinking 4 glasses of alkaline water is much more effective than 8 glasses of regular, bottled water or filtered tap water. There are devices called water ionizers (like a Kangen water macine) that split alkaline minerals and acid minerals in regular tap water by electrical means. Add real lemon to your water and/or put 1 drop of Young Living peppermint oil in your water bottle.
- **Quality Air** - If your environment is polluted with chemicals, dust, smoke, pet dander, mold, and micro-organisms, then much of your energy reserves will be used just for detoxifying. Today, even in the forest and near the ocean, the amount of negative ions are much lower than they were only a few decades ago. Since we now seal buildings to conserve energy and have made our homes and furnishings with synthetic materials, the number of cases of asthma and chronic fatigue has risen dramatically.
- **Food Combining** - Consuming foods in the proper combination is the key to creating an alkaline environment, because when you combine food properly you reduce putrefaction in the body creating a more alkaline condition. Juiced greens, like kale and spinach, are very helpful in filtering out toxins and acidity in the body.
- **Alkaline Diet** - Eating an alkaline diet is powerful in restoration. In general, it is important to eat a diet that contains both acidic and alkalizing foods. For most, the ideal diet is 75 % alkalizing and 25 % acidifying. See the pH Food List on the next page and see Master Cleanse.
- **Green Foods** and liquid chlorophyll offer excellent body cleansing support while providing vital minerals from green alfalfa plants that are easily assimilated by the human body. Drink two ounces of alkaline juice made from organic carrot, celery, kale, spinach and beet once a day or take MultiGreens from Young Living.
- **Enzymes** are essential; without them the body cannot maintain a balanced pH. Enzymes are necessary for proper digestion and support correct mineral utilization.
- **Minerals** - Take a magnesium, calcium, sodium and potassium complex. Your bones are affected by pH more than any other part of the body. Magnesium is a vital element and is essential for over 300 biochemical reactions including glucose metabolism and production of cellular energy, regular heartbeat, and supporting vein health.

Contains excerpts from *Alkalize or Die,* by Dr. T.A. Baroody, Jr

pH Food List

ALKALIZING

VEGETABLES
Alfalfa
Barley Grass
Beets
Beet Greens
Broccoli
Cabbage
Carrot
Cauliflower
Celery
Chard Greens
Chlorella
Collard Greens
Cucumber
Dandelions
Eggplant
Garlic
Green Beans
Green Peas
Kale
Kohlrabi
Lettuce
Mushrooms

Mustard Greens
Onions
Parsnips (high glycemic)
Peas
Peppers
Pumpkin
Radishes
Rutabaga
Sea Veggies
Spinach, green
Spirulina
Sprouts
Sweet Potatoes
Tomatoes
Watercress
Wheat Grass
Wild Greens

FRUITS
All Melons
Apple
Apricot

Avocado
Banana (high glycemic)
Berries
Blackberries
Cherries, sour
Coconut, fresh
Currants
Dates, dried
Grapes
Grapefruit
Lemon
Lime
Nectarine
Orange
Peach
Pear
Raisins
Raspberries
Strawberries
Tangerine
Tomato

PROTEIN
Almonds
Chestnuts
Millet
Tofu (fermented)
Whey Protein

DAIRY
Raw Milk (Goat and Cow)

SEASONINGS
All Herbs
Cinnamon
Curry
Ginger
Mustard
Chili Pepper
Sea Salt

SWEETENERS
Stevia, raw honey, Xylitol, Raw Blue

Agave

BEANS and LE-GUMES
White, Lima and Soy Beans

FATS and OILS
Coconut and Olive Oil

OTHER
Apple Cider Vinegar
Lecithin Granules
Molasses, blackstrap
Probiotic Cultures
Fresh Green Veggie and Fresh Juice
Mineral Water

ACIDIFYING

VEGETABLES
Corn
Lentils
Olives
Winter Squash

FRUITS
Blueberries
Canned or Glazed Fruits
Cranberries
Currants
Pineapple
Plums
Prunes
Rhubarb

ANIMAL PRO-TEIN
All Shellfish and Carp
All Fish Except, cold water fish *

* Better than others in same category

All Wild meat *
Beef
Chicken *
Corned Beef
Lamb *
Organ Meats
Oyster *
Pork, bacon
Rabbit
Salmon *
Sardines
Tuna *
Turkey *
Veal

DAIRY
Butter
Cheese, Processed
Ice Cream
Ice, rice, and soy Milk
Almond Milk

SWEETENERS
Carob
Sugar
Corn Syrup

NUTS and BUT-TERS
All Peanuts
Cashews
Legumes
Pecans

BEANS and LE-GUMES
Black Beans
Chick Peas
Green Peas
Kidney Beans
Lentils
Pinto Beans
Red Beans

GRAIN PROD-UCTS
All Bran
All Oats
All Rice
Amaranth
Barley
Corn
Cornstarch
Hemp Seed Flour
Kamut
Quinoa
Rye
Spelt
Wheat
Wheat Germ
Noodles
Macaroni
Spaghetti
Bread
Crackers, soda
Flour (white and wheat)

FATS and OILS
Avacado Oil
Canola Oil
Corn Oil
Hemp Seed Oil
Lard
Safflower Oil
Sesame Oil
Sunflower Oil

ALCOHOL
All alcohol is very acid

OTHER FOODS
Catsup
Cocoa
Coffee
Vinegar
Mustard
Pepper
Soft Drinks

꘎꘎꘎

Good Blood Gone Bad

Warning: This is a real life story that almost ended in tragedy. I highly suggest that you do not try this for yourself.

Have you ever had a near death experience? Let me start off by saying that this is a very interesting and true story that happened April 9th, 2010. I was on a 40 day Master Cleanse, juicing fast that ended on my birthday, April 9th. I was speaking at a conference where I met a Mycrosipist, who was performing live blood analysis. Well, since I had been on a 40 day fast, I thought,"Oh my goodness let me test my blood." The mycrosipist was quite amazed. She said "you have the cleanest blood I have seen in a long time." She explained that if you are healthy, you should have one (1) white blood cell for every 800-1100 red blood cells. We had a hard time finding any white blood cells in my blood.

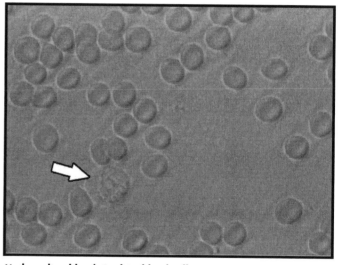

My base line blood, 1 white blood cell.

My mind started to go crazy with thoughts and ideas of what we could experiment with. What would happen to my blood if I consumed something bad? For those who don't know, I love experiments and have been doing them since I have been with Young Living, August 1st 2007. I've even inserted oils via catheter into my bladder.

Previously, I saw in a video that when you use the Valor oil on the bottom of your feet, it will straighten out your blood. I have always wondered if that was true and now I had an opportunity to find out. Then I wouldn't have to take anyone else's word for it.

Someone reminded me that my husband Steve might not approve of this idea. What a way to rain on someone's parade. So I called him and explained my plan, which included coffee. He really didn't want me to do it, but since I don't like coffee, I think he thought, "a few sips won't hurt."

THE EXPERIMENT
Coffee

I decided to do an experiment with coffee. Will it slow down my blood? Is it really acidic? I drank 3 large sips of coffee and waited 10 minutes. I then had my blood tested again… the coffee stopped my blood in its tracks, roping it up and forming uric acid crystals. With that, the white blood cells came to the rescue (5 in one photo slide). I couldn't believe it!

Next, we put Valor on the bottom of my feet and the back of my neck, thinking it would straight out my blood as seen in the Valor "you tube" video.

Ten minutes later we checked my blood again. Shockingly, it didn't change as I had expected. HUM!? My girlfriend, Sharon Schafer was there and suggested I get scanned by the ZYTO Compass Machine. I didn't believe at that time that the Compass Machine really worked. She said, "What do you have to loose? Your experiment is not working out for you." So, she gave ma a scan and it showed that I needed 2 things: Valor Roll-on and Lavender. She applied the 2 oils via Vita Flex on the bottom of my feet and the back of my neck. We waited 10 minutes and then tested my blood again. It was clean! We were totally amazed. I just can't tell you how excited I was to see this with my own eyes.

I called my husband again to tell him what happened and that I wanted to continue the experiments. He objected but I convinced him that everything would be all right.

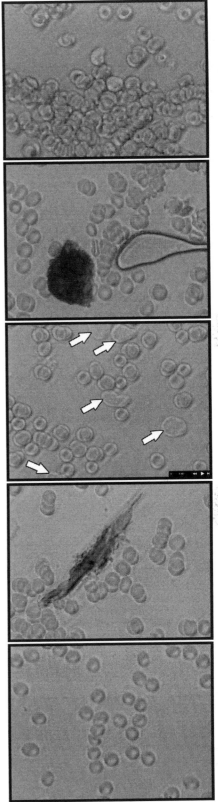

1. Blood after 3 large sips of coffee. 2. Large Toxic Stone. 3. 5 white blood cells in this area. 4. Uric Acid Crystal forming. 5. Blood is corrected after using Young living's Lavender, Valor and Valor Roll-on.

Snicker Charged Candy Bar

On my toxic display rack I had a "Snickers Charge" candy bar. It states "not for children, pregnant women, or people sensitive to caffeine." It is like a monster drink in the shape of a candy bar. I decided to take a bite of that and the Mycrosipist said, "Who only takes a bite?" So I ate the whole thing. With one word in 6 minutes I did not feel good and my legs started shaking, including my thighs. We waited for 10 minutes and re-tested my blood. (The photo speaks for its self).

Now about 15 minutes into it I was really not feeling very well. We used the "Compass" again, which now said I needed NingXia Red, Purification and Eucalyptus Globules. We applied them on my feet and the back of my neck and I drank 4oz of NingXia Red. We waited for another 15 minutes before testing my blood again. It was clearing up, but not perfectly clear.

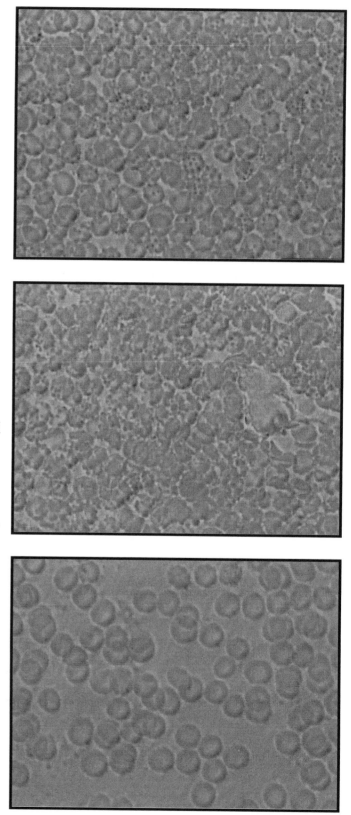

1. and 2. show blood after a Snikers Charge Candy Bar. 3. Blood after the aplication of YL's Purification, Eucalyptus Globules and four ounces of NingXia Red.

Diet Coke

Next, I drank 4oz. of Diet Coke. I use to drink Diet Coke four plus years ago. About 8 minutes after this I started getting agitated and very short on the phone, yelling at my kids, etc. The Compass suggested Patchouli and Thyme and we applied them on my feet and the back of my neck.

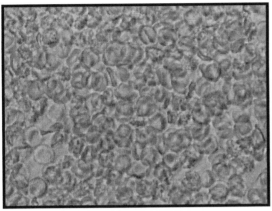

Blood after Diet Coke.

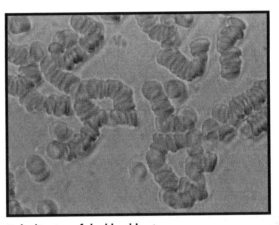

Rulo/Roping of the blood begins.

Fast Forward

After the conference the Mycrosipist came to my home and we continued the experiment for another 1 1/2 days. Everything was working out as I planned. Good Blood goes BAD with everyday products, then we will fix it with Young Living Essential Oils. To sum it all up, this is the total of what I consumed.

- Drank 3 large sips of Coffee
- Ate a Snickers Charged Candy Bar
- Drank 4 oz. of Diet Coke
- Drank 4 oz. of Gatorade
- Drank 4 oz. of Mountain Dew Soda
- Drank 8 oz. of hot water in a Styrofoam cup after letting is sit for 5 minutes (releasing BPA's/ synthetic estrogens)
- Drank 8 oz. of Miralax (Polyethylene glycol 3350 - used as a laxative and before having a colonoscopy)
- Drank 1.5 oz. of Vodka

All of these experiments had dramatic and different effects on the body. Results to the red blood cells included clumpping, formation of toxic stones, and made the blood become staginant. I wanted to do this experiment to educate and prove that YL oils can assist the body in elliminating toxins from our blood.

Effects of the Experiment

In retrospect, this series of experiments was not a good decision on my part. Remember, I had just finished a 40 day fast and my body was very cleaned out.

My body basically went into shock after consuming these products. It took 2 days before I felt the full effects. I taught a class on Monday night and felt fine, Tuesday around 2 p.m. it hit me like a ton of bricks. My old bladder disease came back with a vengeance. Pain came back like it never left, topped with kidney, abdominal, joint and muscle pain which came upon me like I've never experienced.

My left kidney was in severe pain every 20 seconds, it felt like someone was stabbing me with a hot jagged knife. My right kidney pain was occurring about every 12 seconds and lasted for the next 2 days. I began drinking alkaline water, hoping it would flush out my kidneys. I later found out that it was de-toxing my body too quickly. When I stopped drinking the alkaline water, the pain subsided greatly.

To make a long story short, from Tuesday to Tuesday, I was not able to do anything for myself. Per Steve's notes: "Stacey could not stand or walk without assistance, had trouble breathing, talking, urinating, thinking, stomach hurt, no appetite and sleeping. Her resting heart rate was 130 beats per minute, massive head pain- like a band around her head, dizzy, low energy, aches and pains like no other, she officially hated her bed and pillow. She refused to go to the hospital or her doctor, and we didn't have health insurance either." She stated "I got myself into this mess and I'll have to get myself out." I am thankful for my great friends Shannon, Nique and Karen, who came to my home to do raindrop therapy on me. I would hold the Young Living nebulizer diffuser with panaway, frankincense and lemongrass to her nose and mouth, which really helped out with pain, essential oil enemas and rectal oil suppositories. I had learned from of Dr. Youngs lecures the when you use the oils rectal it absorbs through out the body much quicker. She only had 12 oz. of water in a week.

The following are my notes that a friend dictated. As of today, Wednesday, April 18th, I went to a M.D. and got an EKG. It showed that my heart is over working and my resting heart rate fluctuates between 108 – 130 which is affecting my breathing and balance (dizzy), I had to wear a halter monitor for a few days – I have low blood pressure (98/78) where my normal is 120/80. My speech is affected and I have a bladder infection, like back in the day with my IC. I've been dehydrated, as I wasn't able to drink or eat anything due to nausea. I'm glad I went to the doctor today to see what is going on medically – they wanted to put me on heart medication but I decided to treat myself at home without medication. For the last 3 days I've been fighting a fever of 103.5. The fever is currently under control and subsiding.

Overall, on this 8th day I feel much better. I'm using oils to help regulate my heart and I'm actually able to speak full sentences now with improved carity from previous days.

What did I learn? I'm not as invincible as I thought I was! One needs to come off a fast slowly, the above mentioned products really are toxic and can affect our bodies in such terrible ways. If you consume these products regularly they will create inflammation and disease in your body. I have legal size pad of paper of changes I'm making to my home and business life that will be effective the minute I start working again. One of which is I will no longer be working on Sunday. I'm no longer doing experiment with my own body, although volunteers are always welcome! :)

As of today, I will be spending more time with GOD and my family. What I've learned has given me an opportunity to really see what others go through-when people say that they are weak and can't go on – or have to push themselves forward. It gives me a new appreciation of what people go through, as I wasn't able to get my own self out of my bed. I didn't have the strength due to the pain I was having. I'm forming a "Wise Counsel Committee" that I have to listen to whenever, I brainstorm up ideas. I'm continuing cleansing diet nutritional juicing and applesauce, I'll move into shakes when I feel better. I appreciate your prayers and I'm sure I'll be delivered from this shortly. And I am very anxious to get back to my family and to begin helping others in their quest for health.

Keep an eye out for the "Good Blood Gone Bad" DVD for educational opportunities.

THE SOLUTIONS

Take Complete Control of Your Health
Knowledge is a powerful Medicine!

If we take steps to improve certain areas of our lifestyle, a new, healthier lifestyle is assured. Are we eating a healthy diet, getting enough exercise, and quality sleep? What are the consequences if we DON'T change? Weigh the benefits of healthier living vs. the potential risks, such as increased medical cost and loss of wages, inconvenience, or discomfort. Let's make clear, concise, realistic goals to improve ourselves and our family's health and well-being. We must old these habits and decide to start eating a healthy chemical free diet. This could stop and reverse many of the health related diseases like type II diabetes, gout, ADD, sinusitis, asthma, Candida, allergies, prostatitis, pain, IC, MS, cellulits, Methicillin-resistant Staphylococcus aureus (MRSA), eye health, etc.... Our body will naturally heal itself if given the chance.

Eating well does not mean we have to starve ourselves from the foods we love. Our cells must receive nourishment and eliminate wastes. When we start to eat healthier foods we may find that we crave sugar, fat, starch, and processed foods. This is a normal occurrence due to a physiological change in our body's chemistry. During the transition time (30 days), try to avoid sugar, fat, and processed foods. These cravings will become fewer and further between. Eventually we won't crave them or even like the taste of them. Using Young Living Essential Peppermint and Thieves Oil can significantly aid in reducing your cravings for many things.

Even though we discussed this earlier, it is the KEY to your health. Improper balance of acidosis (your pH balance), and candida (an overgrowth of yeast) can create inflammation and disease in your body. Acidic blood can stress the liver and eventually lead to many forms of

Take on a 30-day HEALTH challenge to reverse and restore your health and well-being!

Knowledge is Power!

chronic and degenerative diseases with many side effects. Importantly, too much sugar creates candida and ruins our intestinal tract flora and thymus gland; both control 80% of our immune system. Without flora (good bacteria) your immune system is unable to fight off infection and disease.

Dehydration is another major risk we face today. Drinking fruit juice, soda, milk, or coffee is not a substitute for pure water. All of our body functions need and depend on water! (See pH Balance & Candida Diet chapter).

Those with an acid condition have a toxic liver, meaning they are low in minerals, lack Omega 3 fats, and have an overgrowth of candida. We need to take extra care to eat well. With whole food nutrition and appropriate supplements, you can alleviate many of your conditions. This is good news! Eating raw food will aid in digestion because the enzymes in raw foods are full of antioxidants and photochemicals that help boost the immune system.

Fasting has been called nature's single-greatest healing therapy. It is a great way to jump-start our health and a new healthy lifestyle. A couple of ways to fast can be done by drinking liquid vegetable, fruit juices and/or boiled bone broth. A fast can last one day to several weeks. Fasting can be physically healing while allowing us to focus our energy inward, eliminating physical, emotional and mental toxins from our organs.

When we fast we might feel hungry at times, which signals we need to drink more and start praying or meditating so that our body will heal itself. I just fasted for 17 days and I felt really good, even better than I had felt in a while! For the first couple of days my kidneys hurt, and then it went to my glands in my neck. This indicates that the body is cleansing from organ to organ.

When fasting, the body does not have to use energy to work at digesting our food, which is an all day process. Now our body can use that energy to start to repair itself and clean out stored toxins. In the beginning of a fast, the liver will convert stored glycogen to energy. Then, some proteins will be broken down unless juices provide calories. To be healthy, have energy, and be free of sickness and disease, you must learn to discipline yourself and listen to the needs of your body. I do not believe in water fasting or trying to totally detoxify your body while still eating. Your body functions better while fasting when detoxifying.

Exercise makes fasting more productive, particularly if one is trying to lose weight. NOTE: Pregnant or lactating mothers should not fast. Those with serious health conditions should seek medical supervision before beginning a fast.

It often takes at least 30-40 days to detoxify the body. You can reverse disease symptoms by removing the underlying cause and rid your body of all residual chemical toxins. To help remove toxic chemicals ON and IN your body, start drinking Young Living Lemon Oil and other citrus oils. This will help get rid of the petrochemicals in the body very quickly. Remove all sugar-free products with aspartame and MSG, learn to 'read' the body, begin recording any health changes, restore depleted nutrients, exercise and get plenty of rest, eat 75% raw foods at every meal, drink WATER, WATER, WATER, and pray for guidance and strength. Remember, renewing your body is an on going process.

Cleansing Steps Overview

Bless Your Body and Improve Your Cellular Function - *Cleansing is a serious matter and should not be taken lightly. Always consult your doctor before starting a cleanse.*

Overview of Steps

1. **Changing To Positive Habits** - First and foremost you need to know that YOU CAN heal your body. A positive attitude is everything. You're doing this for your health. Your body wants to heal itself, so give your body permission to heal. Once you learn the basics of health you will be on your way.
   The book "The Real Me" by Sandra Agazzi Chimenti is a must get book.
2. **Toxic Chemical Cleanse** - Don't consume any of the Chemicals on the Cheat Sheet.
3. **Colon Cleanse** - Do the colon cleanse for step 3 if you're extremely constipated. If you have a bowel movement from 3 times a day to once a day then go straight to step 4. Otherwise, do the colon cleanse now, see step 8.
4. **4 day Liver, Gall, and Kidney Stone Cleanse** - This cleanse has a colon flush included, however, don't do this cleanse if your bowels are not moving freely. You will expel liver, gall and possibly kidney stones. You may also expel parasites.
5. **2 day Liver and Gall Stone Cleanse** - This cleanse is designed for those in an emergent situation of Gallbladder surgery and can be done in 2 week intervals.
6. **Whole Body Master Cleanse** - An excellent whole body cleanse. Lowers high blood pressure, cleans out your liver, pancreas, arteries, MRSA/Staph and more.
7. **Rehemogen (Blood Purifier) & (Heavy Metal)** - Use Rehemogin if you are anemic, have sickle cell anemia or kidney issues (dialysis) then follow this protocol.
8. **Colon/Parasite Cleanse** - This is most important as you're doing a final cleansing of the intestinal tract walls. ICP, Comfort Tone and Parafree, all Young Living Oil products can help you with this. Most people have great results using psylium husk (organic corn husks) in lieu of ICP. You need to drink plenty of water with this cleanse at least half your body weight in ounces. If you find yourself constipated, use Smooth Move Tea by Traditional Medicinals or a Celtic Salt Water Flush.
9. **Young Living's 5 Day Nutritional Cleanse or Core Essentials Cleanse** - This cleanse tastes great and builds your body up with essential nutrients and oxygenates the cells. Drink NingXia Red and Balance Complete Shake mix.
10. **Probiotic Cleanse** - Now we need to get the good flora/bacteria back into your intestinal tract with probiotics. Young Living has Life 5, or make homemade Kefir or yogurt.
11. **Bless Your Body and Improve Your Cellular Funtion** - You are now on your way to a healthier, happier life. Do your best not to go back to your old lifestyle. It can be hard at first! If you get sidetracked for a minute don't beat your self up, just get back on track. No mater where we are in life we can always improve upon ourselves in our ATTITUDES, HEALTH, BODY, MIND AND SPIRIT.

STEP 1 • Changing To Positive Habits within 30 Days

Brain circuits take engrams (memory traces) and produce neuroconnections and neuropathways only if they are bombarded for 21 days in a row. This means that our brain does not accept "new" data for a change of habit unless it is repeated each day for 21 days (without missing a day). You can be on your way to a whole new body in just a few weeks. My family wouldn't change back to our old life style for anything now that we feel and see the difference.

1. Positive changes are imperative. If you're trying to change a negative habit, replace it with a positive habit. Focus on one habit at a time. I do not believe we can create our own pain or disease, although I do think we can be in such a state of fear and despair that it can lead to pain. Don't OVER THINK or analyze things, allow your mind to rest. You must believe and have HOPE! Whatever your spiritual beliefs are, they can play a large role in your recovery. For my family, we asked God to change our taste buds to the food that would please Him and heal our bodies and He did!

2. Take on a 30-day challenge. It takes 21-30 days to form a habit. Tell yourself that you're going to do this habit every day for 30 days straight. Remember, using Young Living Essential Oil (YLEO) of Peppermint, Lemon and Thieves can significantly aid in reducing your cravings for many things.

3. Commit yourself completely. Tell yourself, family and friends what you are trying to do and stick with it. This positive accountability pressure will help motivate you. E-mail friends and family and ask only for encouragement. If you have those who will not be encouraging (you know who they are) then don't talk to them for a few weeks. Do NOT allow any kind of negativity, gossip or drama in your life! If the conversation is not encouraging or uplifting remove yourself from the situation! You need to respect yourself enough not to allow others to bring you down!

4. Set up rewards. Reward yourself every week for the first month. This will help motivate you to stay on track. I love amethyst, so I bought myself a rock of it. I told myself that when I get to my goal, then I could take it out of the box and put it on my desk.

5. Plan to beat your urges. We all have unhealthy urges that include smoking, coffee, soda, chips, snacking on junk food, negative thoughts or gossip. Start monitoring your urges, so you become more aware of them. Track them for a couple days. Then write out a strategy plan to beat them. What helps me most is prayer, smelling and drinking the YLEO Peppermint oil. You can also place a drop of YLEO Peppermint oil or Thieves on your tongue, which will help cravings.

6. Track your progress with a journal. Learn to read your body and record what your doing and how you are feeling, including all health changes, so you can see your progress over time. This will help you continue to encourage others & yourself.

7. Most important is to always stay positive. In all things you must remain positive and not get discouraged. Line up all of your thoughts with the word of God. If it sounds like something He would say or do, then be encouraged by that. If not, do not accept it into your thoughts or heart and don't spend any time on it.

8. To reduce degenerative disease, it is necessary to avoid pro-inflammatory foods, cellular deficient foods, Candida, and acid forming foods. All are equally important.

STEP 2 • Toxic Chemical Cleanse

Review the Toxic Chemical Cheat Sheet at the end of this book. Make sure you are not consuming any of those chemicals and avoid the following:

1. Avoid all toxic chemicals in food, drinks, personal care products, baby everything and cleaning products. You even need to check organic products: i.e. toxins, excitotoxins, chemicals, fertilizers, pesticides, polishes, additives, coloring or carcinogens. (See Toxic Chemicals List, visit (LivingAnointed.com))

2. Avoid non-organic foods as much as possible. Cloned and genetically modified foods have no nutritional value: i.e., all corn, soy, canola, cotton, potatoes, dairy and animal products and papaya (only use if they are organic).

3. Avoid all hydrogenated oils and fats, most vegetable oils: corn, canola, grape seed, safflower, sunflower or soy based. Cold pressed olive and coconut oils.

4. Avoid all soy. If you choose to consume soy make sure it is organic and fermented.

5. Don't consume refined, processed, chemicalized sugar products that contain added sugars, especially white sugar and high fructose corn syrup (HFCS); both come from heavily processed sources. HFCS has been known to have mercury in it. An average soda (8 oz.) has 10 tsp. of sugar. In a day it will immobilize the immune system by about 33%, while approximately 30 tsp. of sugar will wipe out the immune system from even functioning that day.

6. It often takes at least 60 days without adding known neurotoxins to detoxify your body, reverse disease symptoms and rid your body of all residual chemical toxins. Neurotoxins are known to cause permanent damage to structures in the brain. They stimulate pain-augmenting receptors within the spinal cord.

   Do not consume any:
   a. Aspartame products (NutraSweet, Saccharine, Splenda, Sucralose etc.)
   b. MSG (Monosodium Glutamate) (See MSG and Aspartame chapter).
   c. ACETONE - found in nail polish remover, ACETYLENE used in gas welders, AFLATOXINS found in peanuts, ALBUTEROL prescription breathing medicine, ALUMINUM/ AMMONIA/ ATRAZINE weed killer used on corn, BENZENE found in gasoline, BUTANE found in lighters, CAFFEINE captopril blood pressure medicine, COCAINE, CODEINE PHOSPHATE used in prescription cough syrup, DEIONIZED WATER/DIAZEPAM the prescription tranquilizer Valium, DIGOXIN heart drug, ETHANOL you drink this alcohol, ETHYLENE GLYCOL antifreeze, FLUOXETINE (Prozac), GASOLINE and GASOLINE VAPORS, KEROSENE, LEAD, MERCURY found in the dental fillings of many people, and HFCS.

7. Alcoholic beverages and all forms of tobacco.

8. Avoid non-organic peanuts, they're high in mold and heavily sprayed with fungicides.

9. Avoid non-organic, tainted/cloned animal products; lard, meat fats and dairy fats.
   a. Cut out all meat (especially salt-cured, bacon, smoked or nitrate-laden foods). Unless your meat is organic, you are eating muscle meat that is fed genetically modified organisms and by-products from other animals. This can include fish, full of antibiotics, hormones and steroids. Watch the *Rave Diet* movie, see the video at (LivingAnointed.com).
10. Fish: only eat wild caught fish unless you know your source. I am down to eating Albacore tuna, (not Blue fin Tuna) and Alaskan pink salmon whether fresh or in a can. Farmed fish: The elevated levels of omega 6 fatty acids in farmed fish keep rising year after year, replacing the omega 3 fatty acids. Part of the reason why is because farmed fish are fed genetically modified soybean pellets that contain insecticides, herbicides and various pesticides. Also, antibiotics are used to control disease and parasites.
11. Don't consume refined processed white flour, glutens, wheat or brewers yeast.
12. The consumption of coffee, caffeinated teas, energy drinks, chocolate, soda pop, and carbonated beverages leads to mineral deficiency. Caffeine also contributes to sleep disturbances, lowered immunity and is the highest acid producing addtives.
13. Stop eating HEAVY meals for dinner, especially meats. Your body needs to be resting at night, preparing for the next day, not digesting food. Eat your biggest meal with lots of protein in the morning; it will give you the energy you need throughout the day. See the Clock Diet chapter.

STEP 3 • Colon Cleanse

Internal cleansing is the key to your health! About 80% of your immune system is located in your intestinal tract. It is imperative to do a colon cleanse followed by probiotics (good bacteria/flora). Waste products and gases in the colon have a high concentration of toxins that may leak into the organs and tissues. When the intestinal walls are caked with hardened fecal matter, nutrients and wastes cannot be transferred efficiently. It is optimal to have a bowel movement after each meal. If your movements are every other day or every 2, 3, 5, 8, 15 days, that is a serious problem. See "How Do You Doo" chart. That may sound impossible, but it is actually a reality for many. If you know someone in that situation please, have them get help ASAP. The Intestinal Cleanse is effective at relieving these afflictions: constipation, chronic fatigue, asthma, flu and colds, allergies, nagging backache, respiratory disorders, digestive problems such as gas, indigestion, and abdominal pain; prostate problems, menstrual troubles, headaches, and skin eruptions.

ComforTone® is an effective combination of herbs and essential oils that supports the health of the digestive system. Its all-natural ingredients bind, eliminate and "scour" residues from the colon and enhance the colon's natural ability to function at an optimum level. Because it supports normal peristalsis (the wave-like contractions that move food through the intestines), ComforTone® is the ideal product for strengthening the digestive system which is ultimately responsible for delivering nutrients throughout the body. It also contains ingredients that are beneficial to the health of the liver and gall bladder.

I.C.P.™ is an advanced mix of toxin-absorbing fibers, including psyllium for the relief of occasional constipation. It also includes a unique blend of therapeutic grade essential oils and fiber. It acts like liquid foaming drain cleaning, scouring your intestinal walls.

Essentialzyme™ is an advanced multi-enzyme complex that promotes complete digestion and assists in the assimilation of nutrients. Enzymes help digest toxic waste and gases from everyday metabolism. They are vital for breaking down proteins and processed foods, which might otherwise ferment and/or rot in the digestive system.

STEP 4A • Liver, Gallbladder and Kidney Stone Cleanse (Option A)
Expel Stones In Just 4 Days!

This cleanse really works! I personally expelled over 100 stones! Austin, my 10-year-old expelled 65 stones and one was bigger than a nickle. Most importantly, I know people who were scheduled for gallbladder surgery and after following this cleanse, they

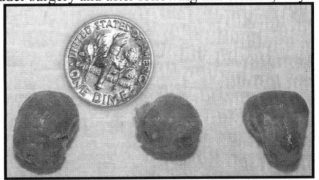

surprised their doctors for they no longer required the surgery! There are a few restrictions to the cleanse: bowel movement regularities, age and health status. Please make sure you read Steps 4 and 5 before you begin the cleanse.

The liver is the largest gland in the body and it's located at the beginning of the small intestine. The gallbladder is located behind the liver near its base. The main purpose of the liver is to produce bile and act as a filter to detoxify and purge harmful chemicals (such as alcohol, hydrogenated oils, high fructose corn syrup, etc.) from the body. Millions of people in the U.S. believe they suffer from gallstone related pain. However, they are, in fact, suffering from liver stones. Liver stones are the less publicized cousins of the gallstone, because the two are essentially the same. Please be aware that even if you do not have a gallbladder you can still expel liver stones.

The gallbladder stores bile created by the liver and releases it through the biliary ducts into the duodenum, to promote digestion. Bile is necessary for our body, especially for fat digestion and the absorption of vitamins such as A, D, and E. The flow of the bile can be obstructed due to liver stones that have made their way down to the gallbladder. The gallbladder becomes inflamed and creates infections with serious consequences. Obstructions can cause poor digestion, jaundice and severe abdominal pain and prohibiting your body from working correctly.

The most common symptoms include chronic gas, belching, pain, bloating, headache, bad temper, sluggishness, nervousness, jaundice and severe pain in the right side of the abdomen under the rib cage.

It is recognized that liver and gallstones are primarily caused by the intake of hydrogenated fats and oils, due in part to the difficulty of digesting these fats and oils. Because hydrogenated fats and oils enhance the shelf life of many products, they are commonly used by fast food restaurants and processed food companies, as well as in the manufacture of drinks, body care products, and even baby formula! Hydrogenated fats and oils have a devastating effect on those who eat such foods. They were toxic before you consumed them, so naturally they create toxicity in your body.

Contributing factors for liver and gallstone formation:

- Hydrogenated fats and oils
- High Fructose Corn Syrup
- Coffee
- Chocolate
- Cola drinks
- Artificial sweeteners
- Preservatives
- Tobacco
- Aspirin
- Salt
- Alcohol

The Cleanse - 4 Day Liver/ Gall Stone

Once again, you should always consult your doctor before starting a cleanse. The side effect of this cleanse is that a stone could get lodged in your bile duct.

For most people, the cleanse is painless. However, permit me to point out that although my husband did not have any problems, I did experience discomfort on my second day for about 6 hours when my stones were awakened from their 'hibernation". I stuck through it and I was amazed to see gallstones on the 4th day! Even suffering this discomfort, the cleanse was worth it because, in a short period of time, I felt

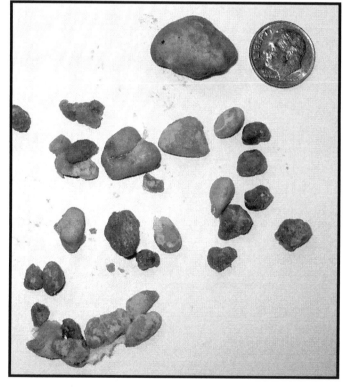

such an improvement in my whole being. You may also experience a headache or migraine which means that your body is trying to detoxify! If you push through, it has been my experience that you will pass a number of stones on the 4th day. It is not painful to pass the stones; it just feels like you're having a bowel movement. Remember, Austin did it and passed 65 stones at 10 years old. He is not a sickly child. It is all due to the poor food choices I gave him from 0-8 years old. Allow yourself 4 days to complete the stone cleanse. It is simple and inexpensive!

Reactions to Cleanse

There is the possibility that during the night you may feel nauseous as well as the need to vomit. This is a reaction to the gallbladder ejecting the stones with such force that the oil is forced back into the stomach. When the oil returns to the stomach you could feel sick. However, there will not be any sharp pain, just a mild contraction. To recover from conventional gallbladder surgery may involve many months of pain and suffering as the scar tissue mends. To help with nausea, rub peppermint oil on your mastoid and over your navel. Additionally, put a few drops in your hands and inhale and/or drink one drop of peppermint oil in 8-10 oz. of water.

Shopping list for Liver and Gall Stone Cleanse - per person

1. 3 gal. of apple juice: try to obtain freshly pressed, raw apple juice or juice your own apples, or bottled unsweetened apple juice, but NO concentrated or artificial sweeteners. *If your in MI. go to AlMAR Organic Apple Orchards.*
2. 4 gal. of steam distilled water (no water containing minerals)
3. 1/2 cup cold-pressed olive oil
4. 1 straw (optional)
5. 6 organic lemons. You will need 1/4 cup lemon juice on the 3rd day and the rest is for what you need on the 4th day
6. Young Living oils: Peppermint, Lemon, Orange, and Juva Cleanse
7. Celtic sea salt or Himalayan salt
8. See Day 4 and Beyond for additional beneficial items.
9. Watch LiverStone Cleanse video on my website to get a better understanding.

Directions: Days 1- 3

1. For day 1, 2 & 3 you drink up to 1 gal. of apple juice/cider and 1 gal. of distilled water a day. You will not feel hungry. The apple juice will give you energy, which you require in order to avoid any fluctuation in your blood sugar levels. The malic acid and pectin in the apples are responsible for softing up the stones.
2. Each morning or evening do an intestinal FLUSH (see options below). This is a important step to do; it makes sure the poisons do not settle in your intestinal tract.
   a. Salt Water Flush: Drink salt-water upon arising. To do this, add <u>2 level tsp.</u> of Celtic Sea Salt or uniodized sea salt (no white colored salt) to <u>1 qt. (32 oz.)</u> of lukewarm water. Shake well, and drink the entire quart. Then if possible, lay on right hand side for 5-10 minutes. This allows the salt water to go right into your intestinal tract and not sit in your stomach. This will flush out your entire digestive tract and colon from top to bottom, usually within an hour, prompting you to eliminate several times, clearing out the plaque and debris from the walls, and the parasites that have been living there.

b. Young Living <u>Comfort Tone & ICP</u> helps keep your colon clean with an advanced mix of fibers that scour out residues. You are supposed to have a bowel movement 3 times a day to maintain optimal health. These fibers decrease the buildup of wastes which improves the absorption of nutrients, which in turn helps to maintain a healthy heart and colon. Take as directed.

c. Herbal laxative: Drink Smooth Move Tea right before bedtime to help with elimination, if needed. You do not need to do all 3 unless you are really backed up. You will have to judge.

Day 3

On the evening of the third day, when you are ready for bed, follow these steps:

1. Drink <u>1/2 cup of cold pressed olive oil</u>. Do not buy the refined oils. You want the oil to be room temperature. You can use a straw to sip it or simply gulp it down, but in order to avoid the unpleasant taste do not allow the oil to touch your lips! You can also mix step 1 (olive oil) and step 2 (lemon) together and drink at same time.

2. Immediately after taking the olive oil, drink <u>1/4 cup of organic fresh squeezed lemon juice</u>. After drinking the oil and lemon, you may feel like burping, or even vomiting. To ease this discomfort, use 1 drop of Young Living Peppermint essential oil. Put a drop on your tongue with a little bit of water or you can inhale it or rub it on your stomach area and mastoid bone. Swishing 1 TBS. of tomato juice in your mouth immediately following oil will help stop the gagging feeling.

3. Go directly to bed and lie down on your right side, this is the most effective position for the oil to do its work. If your position changes while sleeping, that is fine. Put a pillow between your knees may make it more comfortable.

Day 4

Please make sure you're at home on the 4th day as you will be visiting the bathroom quite frequently. It is different for everyone, some start expelling stones anywhere from 8am to 5pm. You will pass stones on the 4th day and it is possible to still be expelling stones on the 5th day. You must do the salt water flush in the morning! When the stones come out you will see lumpy "stuff" in the toilet, the stones can be covered in bile. If you gather them up and wash them off you will see your stones. They will be all different sizes and may be yellow green, turquoise, emerald or black in color.

1. On the 4th day you swich to doing the <u>Master Cleanse</u> (STEP 5). This will aid in healing the Liver and Gallbladder more quickly. Continuing on the Master Cleanse, even for just a few days, will benefit you greatly. I like to ask people to push themselves. If you're feeling good, then try to continue for another day and so on before moving to the nutritional part of the cleanse. Currently, I am on my 31st day of a fast and I feel good, with energy, stamina and healing to my body.

Day 4 and Beyond

After your cleanse is completed on the 4th day and you have expelled the stones, it is advisable to rid your liver and gallbladder of all infection and inflammation. As you can imagine, your liver looks like swiss cheese with some of the stones gone and both it and the gallbladder are inflamed. Now, even though they are inflamed, they are happy to have the chance to work correctly again. Whether the stones are the size of a pinhole or a nickel your body will now be able to repair itself. The best way to do so is using the following regimen.

1. I recommend you purchase Young Living Essential Oils (YLEO) Lemon & Orange and drink 5 drops in 12 oz. of water and 1 drop of Peppermint in 12 oz. of water throughout the day while taking Juva Tone or milk thistle capsules. Juva Cleanse Oil should be taken as well, apply over liver 3 x a day.
2. Inner Defense (Thieves) capsules are a great help to build up the defense in the body as a whole. Take 2 capsules a day for a 2 week period, one capsule in the morning and one at lunch time.
3. There are a number of foods you should start juicing or eating to support your liver, including beets, parsley, spinach, dandelion, carrots, cilantro, broccoli, cauliflower, garlic and radish.
4. Continuing with the Master Cleanse, even only for a few days, will jump-start your bodies healing process. If not as a fast then at least as a daily drink. See Master Cleanse (STEP 5).

Coming off a fast - See Master Cleanse (STEP 5), for how to come off a fast.

This is not the time to do hard physical work. Each morning or evening, do a saltwater flush to help remove toxins that are being released. This is very important, as it flushes out the poisons that have settled in the rectum before they can cause any problems.

Last, but not least, you must change your diet! If you don't you will be in the same situation in a few years. Your body wants to heal itself! If you "eat to live, not live to eat" you will be successful in healing your body.

STEP 4B • 2 Day Liver, Gallbladder Stone Cleanse (Option B)
Expel Stones In Just 2 Days!
This cleanse is for those who only have a few days before an Gallbladder removal surgery.

You should always consult your Doctor before starting a cleanse. The side effect of this cleanse is that a stone could get lodged in your bile duct.

Two Day Liver Cleanse Ingredients
- Epsom salts 4 tablespoons - (this taste NASTY!)
- ½ cup cold pressed olive oil
- 1 large (¾ cup) Fresh pink grape fruit juice.
- Pint jar with lid
- 3 cups distilled water

Salt Flush - Mix 4 tbs. of Epsom salt in 3 cups water and pour into a jar. This makes four servings, ¾ each, of the Salt Flush. Set the jar in the refrigerator (this is for convenience and taste only). Timing is crucial for success of this cleanse. Don't be more than 10 minutes early or late for the timeline below.

Choose a day when you can rest the next day, you will need to visit the bathroom often. Take no medicines, vitamins or pills that you can do without. Eat a no-fat breakfast and lunch, such as cooked cereal, fruit/vegetables, apple juice, bread and preserves/honey or baked potato (no butter or milk). This allows the bile to build up and develop pressure in the liver. Higher pressure pushes out more stones.

1. 2:00 p.m. Do not eat or drink after 2 o'clock. If you break this rule you could feel quite ill later.
2. 6:00 p.m. Drink (¾ c) of Salt Flush. Have a few sips of water to rinse your mouth.
3. 8:00 p.m. Drink (¾ c) of Salt Flush You haven't eaten since 2pm. Don't eat.
4. 9:30 p.m. Get your bedtime chores done, PJ's, bathroom, dishes, laundry, phone calls, etc. You must be in bed by 10:00 pm for the cleanse to work correctly.
5. 9:45 p.m. Pour ½ cup cold pressed olive oil into the pint jar. Squeeze ¾ cup grapefruit by hand, removing pulp and seeds with a fork. Add this to the olive oil. Close the jar tightly with the lid and shake until mixed (only use fresh grapefruit). Drink within 5 minutes. Sometimes if you drink through a plastic straw it helps it go down easier. You may use tomato juice or cinnamon, to chase it down between sips.
6. 10:00 PM. Lie down immediately. You might fail to get stones out if you don't. The sooner you lie down the more stones you will get out. Be ready for bed ahead of time, don't clean up the kitchen. As soon as the drink is down walk to your bed and lie down flat on your back with your head up on the pillow. Try to keep perfectly still for at least 20 minutes. You may feel a train of stones traveling along the bile ducts like marbles. There is no pain because the bile duct valves are open.
7. If ready to, turn on right side. Go to sleep.

8. Next morning. Stones should start to come out. They may look like chunky diarrhea if you don't clean them off. If you clean them off they will be yellowish, green or black, depending on if they are from the liver or the gallbladder. You will need to pass about 2000 stones before the liver is cleaned out. Repeat this cleanse every 2 weeks as needed.
9. 6:00 AM or later. Drink (¾ cup) of Salt Flush. If you have indigestion or nausea wait until it is gone. You may go back to bed. Don't drink before 6:00 am.
10. 2 hours after you drank the first salt flush drink (¾ cup) of Salt Flush, Last one. =)
11. After 2 or more hours you may start with the Master Cleanse for 1 day minimum.

STEP 5 • The Master Cleanse

(Contains excerpts from Stanley Burroughs)

The whole body master cleanse can be done two different ways. First, fasting while doing the master cleanse involves eating no solid food. Second, use the same drink to incorporate into your daily routines to keep your body systems working correctly. Also, it is better for you than other alternative drinks. I highly recommend Stanley Burroughs Master Cleanse. His cleanse is how you should do it in a perfect world. Perfect!

To accomplish this you need to drink 2 tablespoons of fresh squeezed lemon, 2tbs of Grade B Maple Syrup and 1/10 teaspoon of cayenne pepper in 8oz of water every hour on the hour 10-12 times a day, 6 days a week. Once again, this is the optimal way of doing the cleanse. What I have found is that since it is missing the convenience factor most will not do it. Lets face it, most folks work, go to school, run their kids around, cook, clean, help with homework, etc.

So, the following Master Cleanse is designed for the convenience of a busy life style. Make up a gallon of the master cleanse for the day vs. a glass at a time. The Master Cleanse consists of a mixture of lemon juice, maple syrup or raw blue agave, distilled water, and powder or liquid cayenne pepper.

The breakdown of the liver is the beginning of illness. The liver is the toxin filter. When the liver is flushed and starts to detox and regenerate, numerous troubles begin to disappear. You may experience lowered blood pressure, cleansed arteries, restores pH balance and pancreas, loss of weight, increased energy, alleviation of some chronic diseases, improved intestinal regularity which relieves chronic constipation, pain, indigestion, diarrhea, and ulcers, cleared complexion, brighter eyes, increase resistance to infections, enhanced emotional state, and improved tissues and gums. It also helps dissolve and eliminate all types of fatty tissue. Fat melts away at the rate of about 2 lbs. a day for most individuals - and without any harmful side effects. Mucous diseases such as colds, flu, asthma, hay fever, sinus and bronchial troubles are rapidly dissolved and eliminated from the body. Allergies exist as a result of an accumulation of these toxins and they vanish as we cleanse our body. The types of disease which are a result of calcium deposits in the joints, muscles, cells and glands are readily dissolved and removed from the body.

My husband got rid of his cellulitis MRSA infection by doing this fast for 15 days along with NingXia Red and a variety of oils applied topically and internally. Six weeks later he had a full blood screening and all labs came back free of infection - perfect!

Master Cleanse Ingredients

- 5-7 cups of fresh lemons (No canned or frozen). The best way to do this is using a good blender or juicer. If you purchase organic lemons then wash the peel (see Vegetable Wash pg. 113) and juice peel, seeds and fruit.
- 1 1/4 cups organic Raw Blue Agave or Grade B Maple Syrup, not Grade A. NOTE: If you have diabetes or hypoglycemia, use Black Strap Molasses.
- 2 droppers full of liquid cayenne pepper or 1½ tsp. of cayenne powder. Gradually increase if you can (the more BTUs the better). NOTE: if using liquid cayenne, Dr. Christopher's is the best. Dr. Christopher has 2 kinds so if you get the extra hot only use 1 dropper full.
- 1 gal. distilled water at room temperature or as a warm tea.
- During this time you can take your nutritional supplements.

Fasting

It is recommended to do this fast for 10 days, but you can safely work up to a total of 40 days. Set a goal of how many days you think you can do and stick with it. If you are unsure show long you can go, see how you feel, then each new day push yourself if you're still feeling good. You can begin your fast any time of the day, even if you've already eaten. Once you begin however, eat nothing more while you're on the fast. Mix all the ingredients by thoroughly shaking, then drink throughout the day. Consume no other food, but do be sure to drink plenty of water in addition to the lemonade drink. To accomplish this you need to drink 6 oz. of lemon water every hour on the hour 10 times a day. If that is too regimented for you, then just alternate drinking the water and lemon all day. The lemonade drink contains all the vitamins and minerals you need. I personally just did this fast and my goals were 3 days then 5, 8, 10, 15, 20. I fasted for 17 days and I felt great! I was really amazed by my clarity and energy. I still drink NingXia Red while on this cleanse.

Daily Health Drink

The Master Cleanse is great to incorporate in your daily life routine. My family loves it, we make it up the same way just with less sweetner. Just change the name to Lemonaid when you tell your family. It will be much healthier then store bought lemonaid.

Colon Flush

- Salt water flush: Drink saltwater upon arising. To do this, add 2 level tsp. of Celtic sea salt to 1 qt. of lukewarm water. Shake well and drink the entire quart. This will flush out your entire digestive tract from top to bottom.
- An herbal laxative drink, Smooth Move Tea, will help with elimination. Drink this right before bedtime or in morning depending on your work schedule.
- Comfort Tone & ICP help to keep your colon clean with an advanced mix of fibers that scour out residues. Take 3 a day, 3 times a day. ICP provides 3 gm of soluble fiber and is enhanced with essential oils. The fibers work to decrease the buildup of wastes, improve nutrient absorption, and help maintain a healthy heart and colon.

Coming Off A Fast

1. **First Day:** Start with 4 oz. fresh squeezed orange juice mixed with 4 oz. water. If drinking it goes well, drink several more 8 oz. glasses of fresh orange juice during the day.

2. **Second Day:** Drink several 8 oz. glasses of orange juice during the day with extra water, if needed. Make a vegetable broth (no canned soup). Use seasonal leafy and root vegetables such as: beets and beet tops, turnips and turnip greens, kale, carrots, onions, parsley, celery, potatoes, okra, one or two kinds of legumes, squash, beans, a little salt, cayenne pepper, and garlic. (No MSG or hydrolyzed protein). Cook lightly. Drink the broth, eating only a few bites of the vegetables.

3. **Third Day:** Orange juice in the morning. Then eat the soup in small portions for lunch and dinner. No meat, fish, eggs, bread, pastries, tea, milk, or coffee.

4. **Fourth Day:** Orange juice in the morning. Fruits, vegetables, seeds, nuts for lunch with a salad or fruit for dinner. Gradually start eating normally, don't over do it.

This is a brief guideline. Use common sense when coming off a fasting cleanse. Your stomach has shrunk, and is not used to digesting foods, so take it slow.

STEP 6 • Rehemogen Tincture Blood & Heavy Metal Cleanse

This tincture contains herbs that were traditionally used by Chief Sundance and Native Americans for cleansing and purifying the blood. It builds red blood cells and is recommended for any blood disorder.

- 2 full droppers Rehmogen (50 drops) in water 2-3 times daily.
- Blood disorders: Put 2-3 full droppers Rehmogen in distilled water every 2-3 hours.
- JuvaTone with Rehemogen is invaluable.

Heavy Metal Cleanse

Metals such as lead, mercury and cadmium in microscopic amounts can cause severe damage to our bodies. They disrupt normal functions and can cause allergic reactions, fatigue, headache, muscle pains, digestive disturbance, dizziness, depression and mental confusion. Of even graver concern is the metals tendency to accumulate in the brain, kidneys, nerves, immune system, and fatty tissues. Some highly poisonous heavy metals, such as cadmium, can remain in the body for up to 30 years. As a result, they can lead to degenerative diseases including Alzheimer's, multiple sclerosis, and even cancer. Herbs such as astragalus, garlic, sarsaparilla, and red clover have the ability to bind heavy metals so they can be expelled from the body. Essential oils also have a natural ability to dissolve insoluble heavy metal salts so that they can be eliminated. Oils that may be helpful for natural chelation would be helichrysum, orange or lime, cypress, ledum and Juva Tone, the Cleansing Trio (ComforTone, Essentialzyme, and ICP) and Detoxzyme Capsules.

Step 7 • Parasite / Colon Cleanse, Incorporate Step 3 As Well.

ParaFree Softgels Parasite Cleanse: Almost everyone has parasites in one form or another. For the most part, they go entirely unnoticed until they begin to cause fatigue and illness. Pure essential oils have some of the strongest antiparasitic properties known. Some of these oils include thyme, clove, anise, nutmeg, fennel, vetiver, Idaho tansy, cumin, melaleuca alternifolia, ledum, melissa, bergamot, and bay laurel. Using these oils on your stomach, bottom of feet and for the Raindrop Technique really works wonders. The duration of this program depends on the individual.

- Take 3-5 ParaFree Softgels from Young Living. 2-3 times daily for one week. Begin taking ParaFree 3 days prior to the full moon, because the worms are more active. Continue taking ParaFree until 3 days after the NEXT full moon (35 days)

- First 3 days of cleanse - Eat 1 cup of raw pumpkin seeds each day, between 1-3p.m. Pumpkin seeds have been a known remedy for tapeworms and roundworms.

- Day 4-35 - Eat ½ cup raw pumpkin seeds each day, between 1-3p.m.

- Take 2 capsules of black walnut hull capsules each morning only between 7- 9 a.m. as directed. (your only going to be taking 1/3 of what it says on the bottle.) Black walnut is used for ringworm. Purchased at the health food store.

- **Garlic**- Eat fresh garlic each evening. Whatever amount you choose. Must be raw.

- **Pineapple/Tequila Balancing Drink** - Mix one teaspoon to one tablespoon of 100% agave tequila with 1 tsp.-1Tbs. of organic aloe vera juice in the bottom of a glass and pour in pineapple juice, (6 to 8 ounces). Drink between 6:30- 7p.m.

- **Inner Defense** -Take 1 capsule per day, in the morning, for the entire cleanse.

- **Clove Oil** - Put 10 drops of clove in a 00 capsule and take 2 x a day
- After the cleanse is finished, take 4 **"Life 5" capsules (probiotics)** at night on an empty stomach. Continue for 30 to 60 days.

STEP 8 • Young Living's 5 Day Nutritional Cleanse

Facilitates gentle and effective cleansing to improve overall health and well-being. An easy solution for cutting calories without compromising vitamin and mineral intake. It is made up of Balance Complete shake: A superfood-based meal replacement that is both a powerful nutritive energizer and a cleanser. Also, NingXia Red®: Nutrient-infused wolf-berry drink that will energize, fortify, and replenish your body. Also, Digest + Cleanse is a totally unique Purely Oils product. It supplies therapeutic-grade peppermint, caraway, lemon, and other essential oils directly to the intestine in a softgel capsules. This is what I like to end my Master Cleanse with including Step 9 which is using the Probiotics.

You can also just do this cleanse as you desire it sa a gentle, effective approach to cleansing. Many health experts recommend cleansing as a normal, preventive practice, yet a majority of people only cleanse after they are sick or diseased. Young Living's 5-Day Nutritive Cleanse eases the process with a simple, energizing program that helps you say goodbye to the obstacles and excuses that pre- vent you from cleansing. A minimum of four, short, easy cleanses a year with Young Living's 5-Day Nutritive Cleanse and contin- ued nutritional mainte- nance will help balance the extremes of the modern diet.

Step 9 • Probiotic Cleanse

Now we need to get the good flora back into your intestinal tract. We do this with Life 5 probiotics. After you establish your good bacteria/flora you can maintain it with organic homemade whole milk plain yogurt and/or homemade kefir. Both are an excellent forms of probiotics. Life 5 is an unsurpassed acidophilus culture. Each tablet contains acidophi- lus and other vital microorganisms, such as Lactobacillus plantarum and L. salivarius. These friendly bacteria help to maintain optimal intestinal and colon function, and are especially helpful after taking a course of medically required antibiotics. See videos on LivingAnointed.com for more information.

Step 10 • Bless Your Body and Improve Your Cellular Function

Food is the fuel that runs the body. A healthy, fresh organic whole foods diet is impor- tant. Not only will proper nutrition give you more energy and make you generally feel better, it will also help you avoid other health problems. Try to eat 50% to 75% of your foods in a raw state, especially vegetables. Eat foods as close to nature as possible with minimal cooking and reheating. Getting 35 grams of raw fiber a day is very important with countless health benefits: this may lower your cholesterol, normalize blood glu- cose, improve diabetes, alleviate constipation, lower your risk for heart disease, improve weight loss, and eliminate toxins.

1. **Water** - Drink a glass of pure water as soon as you wake up to help flush out what your body is dumping from the night before. Every 2 waking hours drink another glass. You'll flush out toxins and reduce pain. Water is the single most important thing for LIFE and good health. Water hydrates your whole body; organs, brain, muscles, ligaments, etc. Try not to drink during meals; it dilutes the digestive juices. When I talk about how much water to consume, you are not to add in coffee, soda, juice, or milk, just plain water. You need half of your body weight in ounces (+ 20 oz. if you are an avid athlete, ill, fasting or detoxing) in order to maintain a healthy body. If you weigh 180 lbs., divide it by 2 and you have a minimum of 90 oz. of water that you should consume each day. Adding fresh organic lemons or 1 tsp. of baking soda to your water is very beneficial in keeping your pH balance stable, alleviating heartburn, and helping filter your liver, pancreas, kidneys, bladder and intestinal track. See water document.

2. **Breads and Whole Grains** - Whole grain breads have 18 more nutrients than white bread. Check your ingredient labels. Get a whole grain such as oats or whole wheat and not just enriched white flour. Eating 3 daily servings of properly pre-pared whole grains can reduce the risk of heart disease by 25% to 36%, stroke by 37%, and type II diabetes by 21% to 27%. Whole grains include oats, whole wheat, brown rice, bulgur, and rye. Words like "sprouted" or "raw" or "whole grain" indi-cate higher-quality natural foods. Sprouted grains and seeds are far healthier than non-sprouted. Raw foods are healthier than processed or cooked. Eat your foods as close to the state in which they were grown as feasible.

3. **Choose a Wide Variety of Fiber Sources** - Peas, lentils, beans, oats, fruits, whole grains, and vegetables are the best sources. Look for words like whole wheat, hard red winter wheat, barley, triticale, oats, barley, rye, brown rice, buck-wheat, millet, oatmeal, and bulgur. For a snack, eat whole grain crackers, granola bars, homemade trail mix, mixed nuts, popcorn (with unrefined butter and salt), or grab a handful of fiber-rich fruits such as wolfberry, apple and pear w/skin, avocado, papaya, guava, cantaloupe, dried figs, raisins, orange, apricots (dried), mango, strawberries, kiwi, grapefruit, and banana.

4. **Juicing** - This helps you absorb all the nutrients from the vegetables. This is im-portant because most of us have impaired digestion as a result of making less-than-optimal food choices over many years. This limits your body's ability to absorb all the nutrients from the vegetables. Drink 2 oz. alkaline juice made from carrot, celery, kale, spinach and beet once a day. The human body easily assimilates green foods and liquid chlorophyll and Young Living's MultiGreens offers excellent body cleansing support while providing vital minerals from green alfalfa plants. Take a magnesium, calcium, sodium and potassium complex. Your bones are affected by pH more than any other part of the body. Magnesium is a vital element and is essen-tial for over 300 biochemical reactions, including glucose metabolism and produc-tion of cellular energy, regular heartbeat and support for vein health.

5. **Enzymes** are essential; without them the body cannot maintain a balanced pH. Enzymes are necessary for proper digestion and support correct mineral utilization. Organic papaya is a natural enzyme. See Enzyme section of this book.

6. **Broccoli and Carrots** - The families of dark green and deep red veggies are loaded with nutrition. These vegetables are low in calories, packed with vitamin A, high in fiber, and contain the cancer-preventing vitamin beta-carotene: bean sprouts, celery, spinach, tomato, broccoli, brussels sprouts, cabbage, carrots, parsnip, peas, pota-toes, sweet potatoes (w/skin), and zucchini. Garlic promotes immune function and increases energy, destroys common parasites and improves digestion.

7. **NingXia Red (YLEO)** is packed with the nutrients of wolfberries: powerful poly-saccharides, 18 amino acids, 21 trace minerals, 6 essential fatty acids, vitamins B1, B2, B6, C and E, protein, and beta-carotene. Blueberry, raspberry, pomegranate, and apricot juices work synergistically with the wolfberry puree to protect eye health, support pancreatic and liver function while supporting the immune system and reducing inflammation. This is our family's one-a-day vitamin.

8. **Potatoes** - Are inexpensive super nutrient. A 5oz. potato only has 100 calories and gives you a high percentage of vitamins C, protein, iron, riboflavin, thiamin, niacin (which helps lower cholesterol), phosphorus, and magnesium.

9. **Pasta** - Pasta is high in carbohydrates that break down into sugar. When buying pasta make sure it is organic because wheat is heavily sprayed and has high mold content.

10. **Fresh Fruit** - Fresh fruit is loaded with fiber, vitamins, and minerals. The sugar in fruits is in the form of a complex carbohydrate, which is much better for you than refined sugar additives. The highest antioxidant fruits: NingXia Wolfberry, Mangosteen, Acai, Raspberry, Pomegranate, Prune, Blackberry, Boysenberry, Blueberry, Plum, Raspberry, and Strawberry.

11. **Organic Raw Yogurt, Milk & Kefir** - Kefir has the highest amounts of protein, calcium and probiotics, the "friendly" bacteria that help fight illness and disease in your intestinal tract, and it also contains benifical yeasts. You want to make sure that the product you choose has no artificial sweeteners or sugar and that it contains "live" or "active" cultures. Some local farms will have raw organic milk, which is best to drink and to make your own probiotics (Kefir). The next best choice would be store bought organic milk. When it comes to purchasing probiotics, you need to have a high-quality probiotic like Young Living's "Life 5". Whatever kind you get, take **at night** on an empty stomach. It needs to have time to attach and grow in your intestinal walls. Good, active bacteria are necessary to maintain a healthy immune system. Visit RawMilk.org

12. **Grassfed and Organic Animal Products** - Everything is about making better choices. When you eat animal products you want to pick the best possible. The 1st choice is grassfed, 2nd would be organic. Grassfed meat, poultry, eggs, and dairy products are nutritionally superior. Where organic can mean that they are eating grains and not just grass. Both grassfed and organic should be free of pesticides, herbicides, hormones, and antibiotics. I notice a big difference when we first started getting grassfed eggs. The yoke is deep orange this means it is very nutritious. The ones we had been getting were yellow or pale yellow. Look for a Community Supported Agriculture (CSA) in your area.

13. **Oats** - Raw rolled oats are a rich source of protein, and will help lower your cholesterol and normalize blood sugar. A tip: by preparing it with organic apple cider you won't need any sweetener. Even better is to soak your oats the night before, by morning they will be ready to go with no loss of enzymes. (No instant oatmeal). Substitute whole grain flour or raw oats in your recipes.

14. **Fish** - Please check your sources (farm raised or wild caught) and origin to ensure the purchase of sustainable fish with low toxicity. Study upon study indicates that incorporating salmon (wild caught) into your diet reduces blood pressure, lowers cholesterol, and helps prevent heart disease. Higher intake of omega-3 preserves bone density, keeping your bones stronger and protected against fractures. Omega-3's can also be found in sardines, tuna, and mackerel.

15. **Lentils, Dried Peas and Beans** - Lentils are a great source of antioxidants, protein, and of cholesterol lowering pectin. They are a high source of fiber. Beans are a great source of protein and fiber and are extremely filling, keeping you full longer and helping to decrease obesity. Some studies have been shown that eating Lentils may reduce the risk of colon cancer.

16. **Go Nuts** - Nuts are a great source of protein and omega-3 fatty acids. Soak nuts to help digest them better starting the enzyme process. For example, soak your almonds in a bowl of water over night, then rinse them off, pat dry and eat. Note: you will have to eat within 2 days otherwise they start to mold (as they are suposed to). Walnuts have especially high levels of omega-3, which may reduce the risk of heart disease and hypertension. Walnuts, almonds, and pistachios are all high in arginine, an amino acid that increases blood flow to the heart. When it comes to peanuts, they have high mold content and are sprayed with fungicides, so only buy organic.

17. **Breakfast** is the most important meal of the day. Eat fresh strawberries or raspberries. Eat other in-season fresh fruit, raw whole oatmeal, smoothies, or organic plain yogurt (no sugary cereals). Do not consume any sugar or high glycemic index foods. Bread should always be toasted; this changes it from a wet food to a dry food, making it more digestible. As a rule, eating proteins such as beans, eggs, fish, etc., is best for breakfast.

18. **Lunch** should consist of carbohydrates and complex carbohydrates and proteins in the form of pasta (a high gylcemic index food, eat sparingly), mixed vegetables, particularly greens and light meats, freshwater fish or chicken. Drink water with the meal. For the person engaged in bodybuilding, consume proteins before 3 p.m. by eating it at breakfast, mid-morning, lunch, and mid-afternoon.

19. **Dinner** - See Clock Diet chapter.

20. **Oils:** use 1st cold press olive oil or unrefined coconut oil for food, and cooking. Coconut oil is also good for skin and hair care (eliminate all hydrogenated oil).

21. All body care products need to be organic with no added harmful ingredients. (See Toxic Chemicals List document). For my family it was very easy to switch over to non-toxic body care. Just because the label says it is organic doesn't mean it is. Always read your labels.

22. I use only Young Living shampoo for my husband who had very bad dermatitis. After using YL shampoo his dermatitis cleared in one week. Young Living has a wide range of body care products from lotion, shampoo, conditioner, face cream, butt rash, etc. Also, Dr. Wood's or Bronner's Castile soap can be used for hair, body, dishes, laundry, washing fruits and veggies.

23. Young Living Therapeutic Grade Essential Oils affect every cell of the body within 3 sec. to 20 min. and are metabolized like other nutrients. They are powerful antioxidants that create an unfriendly environment for free radicals. They work as free-radical scavengers and prevent cell mutation, fungus, and cellular oxidation. When using essential oils make sure they're for internal use only. (see Everything You Wanted to Know About YLEO chapter).

24. Do not consume: refined sugars, white flour, hydrogenated oils and fats, fried foods, coffee, soda, non-herbal tea, energy drinks, artificial sweeteners, foods that have been: processed or over-cooked, synthetic, chemicalized, fertilized, pesticide-laden, polished, filled with additives, dyes, preservatives, genetically modified or cloned.

25. Minimize stress in your life. Write down a list of what stresses you and then find a way to eliminate or fix it. If you know people who will not be encouraging (you know who they are) then don't talk to them for a few weeks. Do not allow any kind of negativity, gossip or drama in your life! If the conversation is not encouraging or uplifting, remove yourself from the situation! You need to respect yourself enough not to allow others to bring you down!

26. Get enough sleep. It can help ease pain, fatigue, restless leg syndrome, and brain-wave irregularities, which can interfere with restful sleep. Do relaxing activities that get you ready for sleep, such as listening to soft music or taking a warm bath. Use YLEO lavender on the bottoms of your feet or put a few drops of coconut, V6 or olive oil in your hand with 2 to 3 drops of lavender and rub over face and neck. Try vetiver oil on the bottom of the feet if lavender doesn't work.

27. Exercising is crucial. Be as physically active as possible and do flexibility exercises because they are necessary to get rid of acid and toxin build-up in the muscles. Lack of exercise weakens muscle tone, causing less blood and lymphatic fluid to flow through the body and worsening symptoms. Sweating is a powerful way to cleanse your body of toxins. A simple 15 to 30 min. walk outside every day is extremely helpful. Using a sauna, eating cayenne pepper and using Young Living ginger oil on your skin, in your bath, or as a tea is known to sweat out toxins and pesticides. Exercise one hour every day (gardening, shoveling, walking, yoga, etc.) and learn to breathe deeply.

28. Organic Apple Cider Vinegar (ACV) is extremely effective in cleaning out your body's system. It is high in potassium, a natural antibiotic and antiseptic that fights germs and bacteria inside and outside the body. Drink an Apple Cider Vinegar Cocktail three or four times daily. ACV Cocktail - 2 tsp. raw apple cider vinegar in an 8 oz. glass of warm water with 1.5 tsp. or so of raw honey, sucanat or agave.

Other Great Information

1. Return all food products with aspartame or MSG opened or unopened. The grocer can return them to the manufacturer for a store refund. The manufacturer should get the message; so will the grocer. You don't even have to have a receipt. I did this and got $70.00 back in store credit. Then call the company and tell them of your disapproval and that you are not satisfied with their product, they will send your money back.

2. Share with others that we do have options. I am so thankfull that I found out and of all places...while camping. Stand up for what you believe in. We do not have to live in pain and despair any longer. Take charge of your life and health!

Top Anti-inflammatory Food List

- Peppers, hot
- Garlic
- Ginger root
- Turmeric
- Onion
- NingXia Wolfberries
- Acerola
- Curry powder
- Fish oil, salmon
- Parsley
- Chard, Swiss

- Chives
- Kale
- Spinach
- Mustard greens
- Apple cider vinegar
- Amaranth leaves, raw
- Watercress
- Mustard greens
- Lettuce, leaf
- Turnip greens
- Beets and greens

- Pine Nuts
- Leeks
- Collards
- Basil
- Coriander (cilantro)
- Cabbage, Chinese
- Chicory greens
- Endive
- Dandelion greens
- Carrots
- Anchovy

The Power of Enzymes!

Our bodies need enzymes to separate the components our food in our body, so the nutrients can pass through the intestinal walls and be absorbed into our blood stream. Without enzymes, food can't be properly broken down and digested. The intestinal track/ pipes becomes congested/clogged with partially undigested foods that cling to the walls and block vitamins and minerals from being absorbed by the body. This will then turn into toxic waste, bacteria and parasites dump. I recommend watching the movie "Osmosis Jones" great for kids.

Metabolic enzymes are involved in every process of the human body. The immune system, circulatory system, liver, kidneys, spleen, pancreas, and even our ability to see, breathe, and think depend upon metabolic enzymes. Our body produces over 20 different digestive enzymes. A majority of the source of these enzymes are found in fruits, vegetables, meats, grains and other foods. Since most of the foods we eat today are enzyme-deprived, our bodies take metabolic enzymes from other parts of the body and use them to digest food.

Enzyme-deprived foods stem from foods being pre-packaged, processed, over-cooked, synthetic, chemicalized, fertilized, pesticide-laden, filled with additives, and/or coloring in any way. They often disrupt our bodies' systems and create disease.

Gary Young, founder of Young Living talks about enzymes and how important they are to good health. "Enzymes facilitate most of our body's metabolic processes, like supplying energy, digesting foods, purifying the blood, and ridding the body of waste products. They also help to increase resistance to disease, improve hormones, sex, immune system and speeds up bone and wound healing, increases mental clarity, helps digest toxins, break down fat, attach iron to the red blood cells, may help dissolve blood clots, prevent or slow aging, eliminate carbon dioxide from our lungs, build muscles, and aid in many other functions".

Some people say, "Well, I eat 60% of raw fruit and vegetables, but I still don't have a bowel movement every day". If most of the fruit and veggies people get right now are from the supermarket they are most likely full of pesticides. One has to realize that even though it looks like a tomato doesn't mean it has the same God given properties as a tomato after man has genetically altered it and sprayed it with fungicides and pesticides. The enzymes are not the same anymore. Here is a list of better choices on how to eat fruit and veggies in order (raw organic being he best): raw organic, frozen organic, steamed organic, raw regular, frozen, and canned.

Live enzymes are supplied in raw food, but as soon as we cook or process our food, we kill all the enzymes. This is the most overlooked fact in health today. Until this problem is corrected the body will continue to struggle and suffer.

Your health can be determined by one of the two choices:

1. Not taking digestive enzymes with your food will make your body use energy and enzyme reserves to help digest the cooked and processed food. This causes the body to be distracted from its main function, protecting and repairing itself.

2. The best way to take digestive enzymes is before you eat on an empty stomach. This will help to better digest the food. Taking enzymes between meals help clean up your blood. This will conserve the body's energy and enzyme reserves. Digesting your food properly and cleaning up the blood makes it possible for the human body to give all of its attention to protecting and repairing itself. It will no longer have to get involved in cleaning up the blood of undigested particles. If you want a fully functional, effective and strong immune system, then improving digestion and cleaning up the blood is the way to go. This gives the body back its full power to protect and repair. Great health is the most valuable possession a person can own.

Enzymes infused with Young Living Essential Oils.

Essentialzymes 4 - (E-4) is a multi-spectrum enzyme complex specially formulated to aid the digestion of dietary **fats, proteins, fiber, and carbohydrates** . **E-4** combines both animal- and plant-based enzymes into a single solution to help the body more completely break down problematic foods such as high fats and excessive starch. The plant-based enzymes capsule is designed to release immediately upon entering the stomach, where the pH environment is more acidic. The animal- based enzyme capsule is formulated to delay its release in the lower intestine region, where the environment is more alkaline and the pH level is better suited for animal-based enzyme breakdown and proper absorption.

EssentialZyme - is an advanced multi-enzyme blend that aids digestion and enhances the absorption of nutrients. As we grow older, our pancreas produces fewer digestive enzymes, and we become less able to unlock the nutrient content, vitamins, and minerals from our food. Enzymes are vital for breaking down proteins and processed foods, which might otherwise ferment and putrefy in the digestive system. Undigested foods sap energy and promote overgrowth of yeast, fungi, and parasites in the intestinal tract.

Allerzyme - A high-powered enzyme complex of vegetable enzymes that promotes complete digestion of proteins, carbohydrates, and fats. Incomplete digestion can cause allergies and yeast fungus over growth. It is enhanced with therapeutic grade essential oils.

Detoxzyme - contains a powerful vegetarian based enzyme combined with anise seed and fennel essential oils to detoxify the liver and create a healthy intestinal environment.

Mightyzyme - A high-powered chewable multi-enzyme formula for children and even adults. Per Gary Young "babies who are fed formula are enzyme deficient and develop toxic condition, such as mucus, fevers, diarrhea, colic, allergies, mental disturbances, ADHD, and autism.

Candida Diet

Candida (candidiasis) is a friendly yeast (flora) that lives in the intestines. It feeds the good bugs that help our bodies stay healthy. If this good bacteria is compromised through the use of antibiotics, oral contraceptives, steroids, stress, or following prolonged illness, the digestive system becomes unbalanced causing chronic candida. Adrenal insufficiency and diabetes have been cited as factors which encourage excess candida. Also, studies of autoimmune patients have shown that a key factor in all of these serious diseases is an overgrowth of candida. Candida causes dietary allergies that can trigger the symptoms of autoimmune disease upon ingestion. Candida also promotes inflammation. In order to grow, candida makes you crave foods that feed it, such as sugar, carbohydrates, yeast, and pasteurized cows' milk products anything that brakes down into sugar. Candida can even penetrate through the bowel wall, passing into the bloodstream and throughout the body. People with severely weakened immune systems may develop a widespread candida infection. An overgrowth of Candida Albicans yeast in the intestines is responsible for symptoms such as fatigue, headache, mood swings, sinus congestion, depression, poor memory and concentration, and cravings for sweets.

Foods to AVOID on the Candida Diet

Successful Anti-Candida dieters normally report improvements within the first month. It is a tough lifestyle change at first; however, when the Candida infection is beaten, all of the foods to avoid can be slowly reintroduced into your diet. Do not eat microwave cooked foods, as this weakens the immune system. Always drink filtered water.

Dairy - First, reduce or eliminate pasteurized dairy products. Pasteurization destroys enzymes, vitamins C, B12 and B6, diminishes proteins, kills beneficial bacteria, promotes pathogens and is associated with allergies, increases tooth decay, causes colic in infants, growth problems in children, osteoporosis, arthritis, heart disease, cancer and candida. Raw milk, on the other hand, is very beneficial for you. It predigests the protein of cultured milk (yogurt, kefir) thus enhancing digestion, absorption and contains natural probiotics.

Additives, Preservatives, and Oils - If you see something on the list of ingredients that you don't know or can't pronounce, chances are you should steer clear. Non-organic food like meat or eggs can also contain residual levels of antibiotics and steroids that were used during the farming process. These chemicals can disrupt your friendly bacteria and allow the Candida yeast to flourish. Do not eat food additives or processed food. Avoid all heated oils, fats, and hydrogenated fats as these compromise the immune system. (This does not include eating beneficial raw coconut oil. See Healthy Oils section).

Alcohol - Alcohol is high in sugar, which that can feed the growth of the Candida yeast and put stress on your organs and immune system. Wine, beer, etc. are all off-limits, but these can be reintroduced when the diet starts to work!

Caffeine and Other Drinks - Coffee, sodas, energy drinks, artificial sweeteners, sugar, and chocolate kick-start your candida. The level of sugar, caffeine, taurine, guanara, and ginseng in these beverages are so high that no serious candida dieter should consider having any. You may think that sugar-free diet soda is a safe option on the candida diet, but in fact it can feed your candida just as much as a sugary soft drink. Also, no carton or bottled fruit juices, especially with added sugar of any kind.

Fruits - While fruit is good for you, its high sugar content helps to feed the growth of Candida. Avoid fresh, dried, and canned fruit, especially fruits like melon that may contain mold. No over-ripe fruit, bananas, melon, or grapes - the natural sugar levels in these are too high. Granny Smith apples would be ok in moderation. After a few months all fruits may be eaten in moderation.

Note: anything with a seed is a fruit, i.e. cucumber, squash, green pepper, etc., is really a fruit. You can look up the definition of fruit and vegetables in the dictionary or look up cayenne pepper and it will say it's a fruit.

Glutenous Foods - Avoid foods containing gluten, basically anything made with wheat, rye, oats, or barley. Cut out foods like wheat and rye bread and pasta. Some people are very sensitive to gluten; if you're not careful your body will spend all of its time combating these glutenous food instead of attacking the candida. Yeast-containing foods include: Baker's yeast, Brewer's yeast, Engevita, Torula, and any other types of nutritional yeast. Baked goods raised with yeast such as breads, rolls, crackers, bagels, pastries, and muffins are not permitted.

Mushrooms - Mushrooms and truffles are fungi, and candida loves to feed on mold and fungi. It is best to cut them out.

Nuts - Nuts that are high in mold, like peanuts, can promote a Candida outbreak. Stick to freshly cracked or whole nuts. Soak nuts to help your body digest them better. For example, soak your almonds in a bowl of water over night, then rinse them off, pat dry and eat. Note: you will have to eat within 2 days otherwise they start to mold.

Sugars, Honeys and Syrups - That includes any chemical ending in 'ose', like lactose, sucrose, fructose, etc. Sugars feed the growth of your Candida infection. No sugar, honey, or artificial sweeteners (Stevia and Raw Blue Agave are a safe alternative). All candy, chocolate, sugar cereals or bars should be eliminated.

Vinegar - Vinegar is made in a yeast culture, which depletes the stomach of acids and can also cause inflammation in your gut. Although **apple cider vinegar** can be helpful in combating yeast, other types should be avoided: red wine, white, rice and balsamic vinegar. You should also avoid sauces and condiments such as mayonnaise, salad dressing, ketchup, Worcestershire, steak or BBQ sauce, shrimp sauce, soy sauce, mustard, pickled anything, green olives, relishes, horseradish, mincemeat, and chili sauce.

Foods to Eat on the Candida Diet

Vegetables - There are some vegetables that will actually inhibit the growth of candida. These include raw garlic, onions, cabbage, broccoli, turnip, and kale. Keep starchy vegetables like potatoes and yams to a minimum. You should buy your vegetables fresh and steam them. You may add garlic for flavor. Not only do vegetables starve the candida of its sugar and mold, they also absorb fungal poisons and carry them out of your body. Keep **garlic** in your diet; it kills candida. Use fermeted vegetables like saurkraut, kimchi, pickles, etc

Organic Raw Yogurt, Milk & Kefir - Kefir is the best for you in protein, calcium and probiotics, the "friendly" bacteria that helps fight illness and disease. You want to make sure that the product you choose has no artificial sweeteners, is low in sugar and that it contains "live" or "active" cultures. Some local farms will have raw milk, which is better than regular or organic store bought if you plan on consuming a cow's dairy products. http://livinganointed.com/links#co_ops

Probiotics will restore balance to your gut to help it repopulate itself with good bacteria (flora). They are absolutely neccessary after a course of antibiotics has been taken, or when a patient is suffering from candida. Good bacteria will also produce antifungal enzymes that can help fight candida and restore balance to your system.

Proteins - Feel free to eat plenty of high protein meals as part of your plan to starve the candida yeast. Foods like pastured beef, chicken, lamb, wild caught fish, and eggs are all good for you anyway, but they serve an extra purpose in an Anti-Candida Diet. They are completely free of sugars and mold and fill you up while restricting the candida's appetite and growth.

Nuts and Seeds are another high protein option that starves candida. Avoid peanuts as they have a higher mold content.

Non-Glutenous Grains - Wheat and rye are off the menu but there are other grains that you can eat. If you like toast in the morning, try whole grain sprouted or Ezekiel bread instead of your usual brand. Rice is all right for a Candida Diet, but get brown rice or preferably wild rice. For cereal at breakfast, try a low-sugar variety.

Drinks

1. Water is a must, 1/2 your body weight in ounces +20 ounces when cleansing yeast.
2. One drop of **Young Living Peppermint Oil** in a 10 oz. shakable bottle. Peppermint is a highly regarded herb for soothing digestion, restoring digestive efficiency, supporting the liver and respiratory systems, improving taste and smell when inhaled, improving concentration and mental sharpness, and directly affecting the brain's satiety center, which triggers a sensation of fullness after meals.
3. Goat or sheep's milk (dilute sheep's milk 50:50 with water) and their dairy products may be used. Raw Cow milk products such as milk, kefir, and butter are fine. (Kefir is the name for curds and whey in the Bible, very good probiotic).
4. Teas with ginger, red clover, dandelion, or burdock root cleanse the bloodstream and enhance immune function.
5. **Braggs Apple Cider Vinegar** can be helpful in combating yeast. see braggs instructions.

CANDIDA NUTRITIONAL SUPPLEMENTS

- Consume high-potency probiotics to replenish flora (good bacteria) in the small and large intestines, increase absorption of nutrients and reduces digestive disturbances. Young Living's **Life 5™** contains 8 billion active cultures and improves flora colonization up to 10 times. Life 5 builds and restores core intestinal health by providing five clinically proven probiotic strains, including three advanced super-strains to enhance intestinal health, sustain energy, and improve immunity.
- **NingXia Red** is a nutrient-infused wolfberry drink that will energize, fortify, and replenish your body. Rich in wide-spectrum antioxidant activity, it has the highest level of naturally occurring age-defying S-ORAC activity to help support immune function, cardiovascular health, nourish the eyes and it is also an anti-inflammatory.
- **NingXia Wolfberries** (dried) are tasty and good for you. See wolfberryjuice.com
- **Super C™** is a chewable supplement, a delicious way to get a daily dose of vitamin C.
- **Lavender** is the most versatile of all essential oils. No home should be without it. Lavender is an adaptogen, and therefore can assist the body when adapting to stress or imbalances. It is a great aid for relaxing and winding down before bedtime, yet has balancing properties that can also boost stamina and energy. Therapeutic grade lavender is highly regarded for skin and beauty. It may be used to soothe and cleanse common cuts, bruises, skin irritations and is great for candida.
- Candida oil blend of Young Living Oils: **Lemongrass, Clove, Thyme, Oregano, Eucalyptus Globlus, Lavender, Thyme, and Tea Tree.** Apply 3 to 4 drops on your thymus, bottom of feet and 5 to 10 drops on your stomach 2 times a day. Also, make up an 00 size capsule with the above oil and take internally 2-3 times a day.

Top (Fungus) Foods That You Will Want To Avoid

1. **Alcoholic Beverages** are the mycotoxin of the saccharomyces yeast (brewer's yeast). Other fungi besides alcohol can be introduced into these beverages through the use of mold-contaminated grains and fruits.

2. **Corn** is "universally contaminated" with fumonisin and other fungal toxins such as aflatoxin, zearalenone and ochratoxin (Council for Agricultural Science and Technology). Fumonisin and aflatoxin are known for their cancer-causing effects, while zearalenone and ochratoxin cause estrogenic and kidney-related problems. Now, our food supply seems to be universally contaminated with "yellow" corn - it's everywhere! Corn meal, corn syrup, HFCS, our livestock and pets are being fed corn by-products. About 90% of yellow corn is GMO. When using corn products you want white or blue corn and organic is the best choice.

3. **Wheat** and the products made from wheat are often contaminated with mycotoxins. The wheat may be high in mold and sprayed with fungicides. Products include breads, cereals, and pasta.

4. **Barley and Rye** are similar to other grains and can be damaged by drought, floods, harvesting and the storage process. It is equally susceptible to contamination fungi. Barley is used in the production of various cereals and alcoholic beverages.

5. **Sugar** cane and sugar beets are often contaminated with fungi and their associated fungi, but they, like the grains, fuel the growth of fungi. Fungi need carbohydrates-sugars to thrive.

6. **Sorghum** is used in a variety of grain-based products intended for both humans and animals. It is also used in the production of alcoholic beverages.

7. **Peanuts** are highly fungal. A 1993 study, demonstrating 24 different types of fungi that colonized the inside of peanuts used and found the following present; Costantini, A. Etiology and Prevention of Atherosclerosis. This was after the exterior of the peanut was sterilized! Incidentally, in the same study, the examiners found 23 different fungi on the inside of the corn kernels.

8. **Cottonseed** is typically found in the oil form (cottonseed oil), but is also used in the grain form for many animal foods and is often highly contaminated with fungi.

9. **Hard Cheese** will often have mold growing throughout. There is a pretty good chance that there is a mycotoxin not far from the mold. On the other hand, some cheese, such as gouda, is made with yogurt-type cultures. Lactobacillus, and not fungi, are a much healthier alternative.

10. **Common Table Mushrooms Are Fungi.** Naturally, with this list coming from a group that opposes eating food that is merely contaminated with fungi, we'd certainly oppose eating the fungus itself!

The Fungal Etiology of Inflammatory Bowel Disease by David A. Holland, M.D.

Water: How Much Is Enough?

Water is your body's principal chemical component, comprising on average 60% of your weight. Every system in your body depends on water. For example, water flushes toxins out of vital organs, carries nutrients to cells, provides a moist environment for ear, nose, and throat tissues, and lubricates skin, muscles and joints. Without water, we would be poisoned to death by our own waste products. Every day you lose water through breathing, perspiration, urination and bowel movements. People always say, "I drink a lot of milk, juice or soda. Does that count for part of my daily water intake?" The answer is NO! For your body to function properly, you must replenish it with a pure water supply.

When the kidneys remove uric acid and urea, these must be dissolved in water. If there isn't enough water, wastes are not removed as effectively and may build up as kidney stones. Water is vital for chemical reactions in digestion and metabolism. It carries nutrients and oxygen to the cells through the blood and helps to cool the body through perspiration. Most people have no idea how much water to drink in a day. A lack of water will lead to dehydration and most people are currently in a dehydrated state. We even need water to breathe; our lungs must be moist to take in oxygen and excrete carbon dioxide.

How much water do you need a day to maintain a healthy body?

It is impossible to give one-size fits all amounts. There are many variances, but here is a good guideline. The suggested water intake throughout the day is half your body weight in ounces.

- If you weigh 180 lbs., divide it by two, so 90 oz. of water should be consumed each day.
- This guide applies to all people, from children 2 years and older.

Factors that change your water needs

- **Exercising** - an additional 20oz of water is need to keep your body hydrated.
- **Detoxifying** - Add an additional 20 oz. of fluid a day.
- **Environment** - If hot and/or humid or stuck in a heated home during the winter, we can become dehydrated so our body will require more water.
- **Health Conditions** - Fever, vomiting, diarrhea, bladder infections and urinary tract stones can cause our body to lose additional fluids.
- **Pregnant or Breast Feeding** - Additional fluids are needed to stay hydrated. The Institute of Medicine advises that pregnant women drink a minimum of **80oz** and women who breast-feed consume **100 oz** a day.

What other effect does dehydration have on your body?

Water makes up about 80% of the brain and is an essential element in neurological transmissions. Poor hydration adversely affects mental performance and learning ability in adults and children. Memory, attention, and concentration can be decreased by 10 per cent due to dehydration. Symptoms of mild dehydration may include tiredness, dizziness, constipation, decreased blood pressure (hypotension), dizziness, fainting, headaches, episode of visual snow, and a feeling like jet lag, as well as reduced alertness and ability to concentrate. Signs of severe dehydration are increased thirst, dry mouth, weakness, lethargy or extreme sleepiness, light-headedness (particularly if worsening on standing), seizures, sunken fontanel (soft spot) in infants, fainting, sunken eyes, darkening of the urine, or a decrease in urination. These can lead to changes in the body's chemistry, kidney failure, and may be life-threatening.

Always stay well hydrated throughout each day. If the urine is a pale yellow color, it is an easy way to tell that it is sufficient. More water is needed if the urine is dark.

How to perk up your water!

Add flavor and health benefits by adding Young Living Therapeutic Essential Oils to your water.

- Fresh squeezed lemon water every morning right when you wake up to help flush all that your body is dumping from the night before.
- 1 drop of peppermint tastes great and helps with digestion, memory, sinusitis, and headaches, curbs appetite, and freshens breath.
- 4 to 5 drops of any citrus oil -- grapefruit, lemon, orange, tangerine or citrus fresh -- is another way to make a no-calorie, no-sugar, great-tasting drink with many health benefits. Add them to a nontoxic bottle so it can be shaken before you drink it, or get a glass bottle that has a good screw cap on top.
- Adding fresh organic lemon juice to water throughout the day is very beneficial to keeping the pH balanced, alleviating heartburn, and helping filter the liver, pancreas, kidneys, bladder and intestinal tract.
- 2 drops Eucalyptus Globules tastes good in hot water and also is an expectorant, promoting the discharge of phlem or other fluid from the respiratory track. This will rid the lungs of mucus and help alleviate inflammation.

Meatless Sources of Protein
For optimal benefits use non-GMO* and chemical-free organic produce

Row Nuts and Seeds (shelled)

Nut or Seed (1/4 cup)	Protein Grams
Almond	7
Brazil nut	5
Cashew	4
Chestnut	1
Coconut (shredded)	2
Filbert/Hazelnut	5
Flax seed, don't eat whole	5
Hemp Hearts	15
Macadamia	2
Peanut (only if organic)	8
Pecan	2
Pine nut	4
Pistachio	6
Pumpkin seed	7
Sesame seed	7
Soynut (only if organic and fermented)	10
Sunflower seed	8
Walnut	5

Beans (cooked)

Bean (1 cup)	Protein Grams
Adzuki (Aduki)	17
Anasazi	15
Black Beans	15
Black-eyed Peas	14
Cannellini (White Beans)	17
Cranberry Bean	17
Fava Beans	13
Garbanzos (Chick Peas)	15
Great Northern Beans	15
Green Peas, whole	9
Kidney Beans	15
Lentils	18
Lima Beans	15
Mung Beans	14
Navy Beans	16
Pink Beans	15
Pinto Beans	14
Soybeans (organic only)	29
Split Peas	16

Grains (cooked)

Grain (1 cup)	Protein Grams
Amaranth	7
Barley, pearled	4 to 5
Barley, flakes	4
Buckwheat	5 to 6
Cornmeal (fine grind)	3
Cornmeal (polenta, coarse)	3
Millet, hulled	8.4
Oat	6
Oat, bran	7
Quinoa	5
Rice, brown	3 to 5
Rice, white	4
Rice, wild	7
Rye, berries	7
Rye, flakes	6
Spelt, berries	5
Triticale	25
Wheat, whole berries	6 to 9
Couscous, whole wheat	6
Wheat, bulgur	5 to 6

Hot Cereal (cooked)

Cereal	Cup	Protein Grams
Arrowhead Mills Corn Grits	1/4	3
Bob's 10 Grain	1/4	6
Bob's Kamut	1/4	5
Bob's Whole Grain Wheat	1/4	5
Cream of Rye	1/3	5
Kashi	1/2	6
Quinoa Flakes	1/3	3
Roman Meal Hot Cereal	1/3	5
Wheatena	1/3	5

Nut Butters

Nut or Seed (2 Tablespoons)	Protein Grams
Almond	5 to 8
Cashew	4 to 5
Peanut	7 to 9
Sesame Tahini	6
Soy Nut (only if organic and fermented)	6 to 7

Fruits (cooked)		
Fruit	Serving	Protein Grams
Apple	2 per lb.	0
Apricot	med.	0
Avocado	med.	4
Banana	1	1 to 2
Blackberry	cup	2
Blueberry	cup	1
Boysenberry	cup	1
Cantaloupe	cup	1
Cherry	cup	1
Cranberry	cup	0
Currant	cup	2
Date (pitted)	1/4 cup	1
Durian	1 cup	4
Fig	1	0
Grape	cup	1
Grapefruit	1/2	1
Guava	med.	1
Honeydew	cup	1
Jackfruit	cup	2
Kiwi	large	1
Lemon	1	1
Lime	1	0
Loganberry	cup	1.4
Mango	1	1
Mulberry	cup	2
Nectarine	1	1
Orange	1	1
Papaya	cup	1
Passionfruit	1	0
Peach	1	1
Pear	1	1
Persimmon	1	0
Pineapple	cup	1
Plum	1	1
Pomegranate	1	1.5
Pomelo	1/2	2.3
Quince	med.	.4
Raspberry	cup	1
Rhubarb	cup	1
Sapote	med.	5
Star Fruit	cup	1
Strawberry	cup	1
Tangerine	med.	1
Watermelon	cup	1
Wolfberry, NingXia	cup	32

Grains (cooked)		
Vegetable	Serving	Protein Grams
Artichoke	medium	4
Asparagus	5 spears	2
Beans, string	1 cup	2
Beets	1/2 cup	1
Broccoli	1/2 cup	2
Brussels Sprouts	1/2 cup	2
Cabbage	1/2 cup	1
Carrot	1/2 cup	1
Cauliflower	1/2 cup	1
Celery	1 cup	1
Chard, Swiss	1 cup	3
Collards	1 cup	4
Corn, Sweet	1 large cob	5
Cucumber	1 cup	1
Eggplant	1 cup	1
Fennel	1 med. bulb	3
Kale	1 cup	2.5
Kohlrabi	1 cup	3
Leeks	1 cup	1
Lettuce	1 cup	1
Okra	1/2 cup	1
Onion	1/2 cup	1
Parsnip	1/2 cup	1
Peas	1/2 cup	4
Peppers, bell	1/2 cup	1
Potato, baked with skin	2 x 4	5
Potato, boiled with skin	1/2 cup	1
Radish	1 cup	1
Rhubarb	1 cup	1
Rutabaga	1 cup	2
Spinach	1 cup	1
Squash	1 cup	2
Sweet Potato	1 cup	3
Tomato	1 medium	1
Turnip	1 cup	1
Wolfberry, NingXia	cup	32

*GMO: Genetically Modified Organism

**Those taking prescription drugs should check with their doctor, as these interfere with some medications

For more information, see:

www.vegparadise.com

LivingAnointed.com

The Clock Diet

The world's greatest health secret! The Clock Diet was originated by Dr. Charlotte Holmes who maintained a private practice even at the age of 100 years in 1989. This diet was based on the fact that stomach acid and enzyme production (pepsin and hydrochloric acid which is made by the liver) begins in the morning about six o'clock and tapers off during the afternoon hours between 1:00 and 3:00. This diet works by correcting principles or natural law and works for everyone. Any person that habitually and consistently violates the principles of the Clock Diet will eventually suffer the consequences of ill health; physical, emotional, or both, at some time in the future. Sickness and disease is skyrocketing, and just changing to the Clock Diet can have extremely beneficial results in healing your body. The Clock Diet is the greatest single tool with the greatest benefit in health restoration that my family has found. This Clock Diet principle should be the foundation of any health program, no matter what you are dealing with and no matter what you have been taught in the past about your health and diets.

This diet mandates that we should eat our animal and plant protein foods when the enzyme and stomach acid production is the highest so they can be properly digested. It is the highest in the early morning hours only if you had a good nights sleep and you did not eat any animal meats or heavy plant protein foods at least 8 hours before you went to bed the night before. If you ate a heavy protein-rich meal in the late afternoon when your stomach acid production was low, you did not digest the food properly, which then kept you from resting in a deep sleep, but rather just a light but sluggish sleep causing gas created by food fermentation. Now you feel more tired than you did before you went to bed. When you have proteins digesting when you should be sleeping, it restricts HGH production, which is called the WELLNESS HORMONE.

This is the SECRET to this diet! You greatly increase HGH production the natural way by going to bed on an empty stomach, although some people with health concerns may need to eat before bed. Moreover, if you eat a heavy meal the evening before, the liver does not properly create the acids and enzymes for the next morning's heavy meal because it was under stress that night. The liver creates these digestive acids when you are sleeping only if the stomach and intestines are completely empty and resting. All your waste from the previous day should be down in the colon and ready to be eliminated the next morning upon rising. If you have food in the stomach and intestines at night, the liver will not properly create the enzymes and acids for the next morning. Not only this, you are laying the breeding grounds for parasites, fungus and bacteria. Also, when you eat heavy proteins when the stomach acids are low, a lot of undigested proteins enter the bloodstream which then turn into uric acid which binds calcium into stones in your kidneys, pancreas, liver and gallbladder. This also causes hardening of the arteries. In the afternoon you should be eating fruits and complex carbohydrates and leafy green vegetables. Never eat sugar fruit before noon. This causes candida and yeast problems caused by low thyroid. Eat your beans, grains and meats instead.

THINGS TO REMEMBER

- Never eat any food 3 hours before bedtime.
- It is not just what you eat but when you eat it that counts when it comes to overall health. Each one of us has a built-in body clock that affects our sleeping patterns, metabolism, appetite and energy levels. By eating regularly, timing your meals to suit your body clock and getting the right balance of nutrients at each meal, you'll work with the natural chemical reactions in your body that help regulate and control feelings of hunger, fullness, and our inner and outer well-being.
- Many sleeping problems such as sleeplessness, dreams, and restlessness can be overcome quite easily when the Clock Diet is practiced consistently.
- Be patient. It may take a few weeks until you notice a difference in your inner and outer well-being.

A Guide To Natural Sweeteners

"Natural sweeteners" describe sweet foods from which the nutrients have not been removed using excessive temperatures or by other refining processes. Always get raw, organic, unprocessed products.

Raw Honey is obtained by extraction, settling or straining *without* heat, and is loaded with amylases (enzymes that digest carbohydrates) and all the nutrients found in plant pollens. It is an ideal sweetener for porridge and toast, because the amylases help digest grains. Honey does not upset blood sugar levels and contains trace amounts of several vitamins and minerals as well as several compounds thought to function as antioxidants. The word "honey" appears 61 times in the Bible. Raw honey should NOT be given to children under 2 years of age because they lack sufficient stomach acid to deactivate bacteria spores. Only purchase raw honey that has not been fed sugar water. Asking the farmer is best.

Agave Nectar is a low-glycemic sweetener produced from organically grown and processed blue agave plants (tequila cactus plant). It doesn't spike blood sugar levels, with a glycemic index of 11-26. Young Living has the best agave. Otherwise get raw blue agave. It is the preferred sweetener since you don't need much 1/2c. = 1c. of sugar.

Blackstrap Molasses provides many nutrients like manganese, copper, iron, calcium, potassium, magnesium, vitamin B6, and selenium is ideal for those with diabetes or hypoglycemia.

Sucanat is dehydrated cane juice and is rich in minerals, notably silica. It is the best sweetener for cookies and cakes. In large amounts sucanat can upset the body's chemistry as much as sugar. Sucanat is generally available in the bulk bins of health food shops. Beware of a packaged product labeled "sucanat sugar" that is merely crystalline sugar.

Date Sugar is a very nutritious sweetener made from dehydrated dates. It is a good sweetener for hyperactive children because it is high in tryptophan, an amino acid that has a calming effect. Date sugar is delicious on porridge, but it does not dissolve easily, so it is not the best for many desserts.

Stevia is a plant that is 300 times sweeter than sugar, does not impact blood sugar and has zero calories. It can have an aftertaste, if someone is used to artificial sweeteners.

Raw Maple Syrup (Grade B) is made from the concentrated sap of large deciduous trees. Maple syrup is rich in trace minerals brought from below the ground by deep tree roots. Unfortunately, formaldehyde is used in the production of most *commercial* maple syrup, so purchase syrup that is formaldehyde-free.

Xylitol almost gets a perfect score. It is all natural, tastes like sugar, is good for your teeth, and doesn't spike blood sugar levels. Xylitol is a naturally occurring sweetener found in the fibers of many fruits and vegetables, and is extracted from corn fiber, birch, raspberries, and plums.

Organic Crystallized Cane Sugar is not genetically modified or engineered. It is much better for you to use this in lieu of white or brown refined sugar.

Coconut & Olive Oil - A Healthier Choice

All refined oils available on the grocery shelf are as bad as hydrogenated oils. They are loaded with trans-isomers. *Refined* means that the oil has been chemically treated and they are commonly regarded as lower quality. There are many health concerns associated with the hydrogenation of unsaturated fats to produce saturated fats and trans fats by forcing hydrogen gas into oil at high pressure. Both animal and vegetable fats can be hydrogenated, which means they are synthetic. Always purchase **organic first cold pressed and/or unrefined oils, some times it will say just cold press and that is good.**

Coconut Oil

Coconut oil is a highly beneficial healthy fat, but does not actually contain Omega-3 fatty acids. Coconut oil is, rather, one of the best sources of medium chain fatty acids. I'm sure you have heard that coconut oil is high in saturated fats, artery clogging and dangerous to ingest. The truth is, the medium chain fatty acids (MCFA) found in coconut oil are rare in nature and highly health beneficial. MCFA are digested by the body in a different way than the common long chain fatty acids found in most other foods that increase body fat and arterial plaque. MCFA are quickly digested and producing energy. About 50% of the MFCA in coconut oil is lauric acid, which strengthens the immune system and is also found in human breast milk. Caprylic acid and capric acid are also present, contributing to coconut oil's antifungal, antiviral and antibacterial properties.

Organic centrifuged or **Cold Pressed, unrefined** coconut oil is a healthy, unprocessed oil that may help promote balanced cholesterol levels, thyroid function, aids in weight loss, reduces risk of heart disease and other diseases, and helps those suffering with diabetes, thyroid disease, and chronic fatigue. It can improve Crohn's disease, IBS, and other digestive disorders, and it boosts daily energy. It can rejuvenate skin, clear up liver spots and prevent wrinkles.

Coconut oil has been found to have remarkable physiological effects. It is antihistamine, anti-infectious, antiseptic, boost immune system, a glucocorticoid antagonist, and is a nontoxic anticancer agent. When fat isn't formed from carbohydrates, the sugar is available for use or for storage as glycogen. Therefore, shifting from unsaturated fats to coconut oil involves several anti-stress processes thus reducing our need for the adrenal hormones.

In the past, coconut oil had been mistakenly considered unhealthy; however, coconut oil is cholesterol free and rich in (MCFA) "good fats". When you look at the population in the Pacific Islands such as Hawaii, you find one of the lowest cholesterol levels and lowest incidence of heart disease in the world. These people have always used un-hydrogenated, cold pressed, unrefined coconut oil.

How to Consume Coconut Oil – I don't mind eating coconut oil by the spoonful, but I can't get my husband or kids to do that. So I mix tangerine YLEO with coconut oil in a cookie sheet and put in the freezer, then break into pieces and eat out of the freezer when you want a snack. It really does taste good. Coconut oil has a very mild coconut flavor. Coconut oil can be a clear liquid when placed in the sun or in a warm area of your home or when cooking. When below 78 degrees it will be a white soft or solid form. The beneficial fats will not be compromised by heat. You can put some coconut oil in a smoothie on toast and popcorn. Coconut it is an excellent addition to almost any recipe you can replace butter, hydrogenated oils and partially hydrogenated oils. We consume about 3 tablespoons a day. One day try GHEE, organic clarified butter and coconut oil. Greenpastures.org

External Uses for Coconut Oil – Coconut is a versatile beauty miracle, not only does it moisturize skin and help prevent wrinkles, the anti-fungal properties can even improve issues like and athlete's foot and thrush. I love to use it as my face or body lotion by putting some in my hand and a few drops on my Young Living Essential Oil. Mix together and rub over my face and body.

It is the best thing you can use on African-American hair, textured, curly, thick, course hair, or black or gray hair is coconut oil! Use a small amount as a replacement for hair grease or leave in conditioners. It is a good nourishing fats that your hair and scalp needs.

Olive Oil

The best olive oil is **1st cold-pressed**, a chemical-free process that involves only pressure, producing a natural level of low acidity. *It's the finest and fruitiest of the olive oils and is the most expensive.* Olives are a fruit *(Olea europaea),* a traditional tree crop of the Mediterranean Basin. It is commonly used in cooking, cosmetics, pharmaceuticals, soaps and anointing. Olive oil is considered a healthy oil because of its high content of mono-unsaturated fat (mainly oleic acid) and polyphenols. Studies have found that consumption of olive oil can lower the risk of coronary heart disease by reducing blood cholesterol levels and blood clot formation, reduce risk of some cancers (breast cancer), and diabetes. It contains many antioxidant phytochemicals that have many health benefits.

Because olive oil is unlikely to cause allergic reactions, it is used in the preparation of lipophilic drug ingredients. It does have demulcent properties (an agent that forms a soothing film over a mucus membrane, relieving minor pain and inflammation of the membrane) and is a mild laxative. It can also be used at room temperature as an ear wax softener. **Never use olive oil on medium or high heat, as it changes the molecular structure making it toxic. It has the best health effects when you consume it unheated in its natural state such as a salad dressing.**

Olive oil was widely known and used during most of Bible history. It had a wide variety of applications and was a valuable commodity. It was used for anointing the living and the dead, for sacred offerings, for lighting lamps, cooking, medicines, personal grooming, and was also used figuratively for the Holy Spirit.

Toxic Free Cleaning Products

Conventional cleaning products contain harsh chemicals that can affect you, your family, and the environment. One of the easiest ways to protect your family is to stop using commercial cleaning products and start making your own or buying a nontoxic cleaner. In fact, doing so is easy, far less expensive, and just as effective. There are an astonishing number of simple, easy, and affordable ways that basic home ingredients like baking soda, lemon, vinegar, and essential oils can be used to clean, disinfect, and deodorize. The anti-bacterial properties of essential oils can effectively promote greater hygiene, and kill bacteria, germs, mold and fungus.

A portable hot water steamer works exceptionally well for cleaning anything, taking off wallpaper, metal filters, etc. It is worth the money to invest in one. Just be careful; it does get very hot.

Ingredients

- **Essential Oils (YLEO)** - I only use Young Living Therapeutic Grade Essential Oils. Since I will be touching and inhaling them, I want to make sure they are pure and unadulterated. YLEO are less allergenic than synthetic fragrances. (If toxic when taken orally, it will also be toxic when applied topically.) They add a pleasing fragrance, disinfect, kill bacteria, mold, and fungus and promote greater hygiene. Use YLEO rosemary with lemon, eucalyptus globulus, and lavender. Blends: lavender with Purification.

- **Baking Soda** is an excellent scouring powder that can be used for cleaning, deodorizing, removing stains, softening fabrics, and clearing drains. It softens water to increase the sudsing and cleaning power of soap. It is slightly alkaline (its pH is around 8.1; 7 is neutral), so it neutralizes acid-based odors in water, and absorbs odors from the air (trash or refrigerator). When turned into a paste with water, you can rub it to polish silver. For dog and cat urine, alternate sprinkling baking soda (which will neutralize acid odors) with white distilled vinegar. Let it sit for a few hours before sweeping up.

- **Distilled White Vinegar** - There are many kinds of vinegar. What you want for cleaning is distilled white vinegar, which has been purified, so it leaves no residue and has little taste. It is also inexpensive.

EVERYDAY CLEANERS- Homemade

Below, you will find recipes for kitchen, bathroom, and living room cleaners, metal polishes, air fresheners, floor and carpet cleaners, laundry and mold cleaners. Be sure to label your mixtures to avoid confusion. The amounts don't have to be perfect; only make what you need.

- **Air Freshener** - Vinegar and baking soda are great room fresheners. Vinegar deodorizes, while baking soda absorbs odors. A simple recipe of 1 tsp. baking soda, 1 tsp. vinegar (or lemon juice) and 2 cups hot water in a spray bottle can be spritzed in the air to remove odors. Or use YLEO Thieves Essential Oil Blend Spray. The best thing to do is get a glass nebulizer essential oil diffuser. It works great and you can even put it on a house timer.
- **Creamy Soft Scrub** - Mix 2 cups baking soda, 1/2 cup Dr. Bronner's Liquid Castile soap with 5 drops essential oil. Mix together and store in a sealed glass jar. It has a shelf life of 2 years. Use this soft scrub on kitchen counters, stoves, and bathroom sinks. Tip: For tough jobs, spray with vinegar first, let sit, and follow with the scrub.
- **Disinfectant** - In a spray bottle, add 30 drops of an essential oil to 4 oz. of water and 4 oz. of distilled white vinegar. YLEO lemon and other citrus oils are naturally antibacterial and antiseptic. Cinnamon can be used as an anti-fungal, antiviral, and antimicrobial, too. You can even mix them together.
- **All-Purpose Disinfectant** - Add 2 cups of white distilled vinegar to 2 cups of water, 20 drops of essential oil and a dab of Dr. Bronner's Liquid Castile Soap to a spray bottle. Shake well. You can also use Thieves Essential Oil Blend Cleaner.
- **Distilled White Vinegar** - Use to remove grease, wax, dirt, and to freshen surfaces. Vinegar kills 99% of bacteria, 82% of mold, and 80% of germs (viruses). It is also good for taking stains out of carpets, dishes, clearing drains, and as a fabric softener for your laundry. Distilled white vinegar has a scent when it is wet, but when dry it leaves no odor. Spray straight white vinegar on poison ivy to kill it.
- **Dr. Woods, Kirt or Dr., Bronner's Liquid Castile Soap** - has a coconut base. This is a good alternative to petroleum-based soaps. Buy on-line or at the health food store (costs more).
- **Dry Soft Scrubs** - can be made with baking soda with 10 to 15 drops of essential oil to scent (optional).
- **Hydrogen Peroxide or Lemon** - Use as an alternative to bleach.
- **Isopropyl Alcohol (Rubbing Alcohol)** - Put on a cotton ball to remove permanent marker, disinfect doorknobs, telephones, counter tops, or other surface. Don't use on wood - it will dry it out.
- Use **Lemon** or another YLEO citrus oil to take gum, tape, or glue off anything.
- **Lemon Juice** - An excellent cleaning agent on its own, it can also add a nice, clean smell to your homemade cleaners. Lemon juice cuts through grease and stains on mirrors, dishes and pots. Cut a lemon in half and rub around to clean a surface.
- **Windows** - Add 2 cups of distilled white vinegar to 2 cups of water and, 20 drops of essential oil to a spray bottle. Shake well.

Thieves Household Cleaner Proportions Guide

Young Living makes Thieves Household Cleaner. I recommend it highly. NOTE: one capful cleaner = 1/2 Tbs. = 1 1/2 tsp.

- **Light Degreasing** (1:60) - 1 capful cleaner to 3 3/4 cups water
  1 bottle makes 30 qts. of light degreaser (32¢/qt)
- **Medium Degreasing** (1:30) - 1 capful cleaner to a little less than 2 cups water
  1 bottle makes 15 qts. of medium degreaser (64¢/qt)
- **Heavy Degreasing** (1:15) - 1 capful cleaner to a little less than 1 cup water
  1 bottle makes 7, 1/2 qts. of heavy degreaser ($1.27/qt)
- **Pots & Pans** (1:100) - 1/2 capful cleaner to 3+ cups water
  1 bottle makes 50 qts. of dishwasher liquid (19¢/qt)
- **Floors** (1:100) - 1 capful cleaner to 6 1/4 cups water
  1 bottle makes 50 qts. of floor cleaner (19¢/qt)
- **Walls** (1:30) - 1 capful cleaner to a little less than 2 cups water
- **Fabrics, Carpet Spotting, ect.** (1:40) - 1 capful cleaner to 2 cups water
- **Carpet** (1:100) - 1 capful cleaner to 6 1/4 cups water

BATHROOM CLEANER

- Sprinkle the toilet bowl with baking soda, drizzle with vinegar, let soak for at least 30 min. (or overnight) and scrub with a toilet brush; or put ¼ cup borax in the toilet bowl and let sit for at least 30 min. Swish with a toilet brush and then scrub. A few drops of pine oil can be added for increased disinfecting.
- **Shower Curtain** - Plastic shower curtains can mold quickly. Try soaking your plastic lining in salt water. Fill your tub with a solution of 3 Tbs of pure (unionized) sea salt per 1 gal. of water. Do not rinse, and hang curtain: the invisible coat of sodium crystals will seal the gaps in the fibers, preventing mildew from clinging to the material.
- **Mold** - If you discover mold and mildew in your house, first find the source of moisture and stop it. Since mold spores can be inhaled, wear gloves and a face mask. Use a stiff brush or toothbrush, a non-ammonia detergent, and hot water to scrub mold off of non-porous surfaces. You can also use a paste of baking soda and Thieves (kills black mold). Don't rinse. If mold or mildew is present, pretreat the area with hydrogen peroxide, or use Thieves Essential Oil Blend Cleaner. (Do NOT use bleach)

KITCHEN

- **Ovens** - Sprinkle baking soda onto the bottom of the oven. Squirt with enough water that the baking soda is damp. Leave overnight. Rinse with water and a little lemon for a fresh scent. Or spray Thieves full strength and let set overnight.
- **Microwave Ovens** - You can use any general purpose cleaner. Please be aware that the microwave oven destroys vitamins, minerals, enzymes, fiber, strips the nutrients and omits radioactive rays even after you're done using it.

- **Cutting Boards** - Spray vinegar, YLEO Lemon or Thieves cleaner on the cutting board. Let sit ½ hour.
- **Dishwater** - The antibacterial properties of essential oils can effectively promote greater hygiene. Add a couple drops of Melrose or Lemon to dishwater for clean dishes and a great smelling kitchen.
- **Dishwasher** - 2 capfuls of Thieves Cleaner mixed with 2C. baking soda. Put 1tbs of mix in both holes
- **Drain Cleaner** - To clean drains or clear clogs, pour 1/4 cup of baking soda down them followed by ½ cup of white vinegar. Cover drain and sink overflow, vent until fizzing stops, then flush with HOT water. Remove hair from drain and/or use a plunger if needed.

LAUNDRY

- **Laundry Detergent** - Mix equal parts of baking soda and Borax. One cap of Thieves Cleaner and 1/2 cup baking soda can also be used.
- **Fabric Rinse** - Add 1/4 cup of vinegar or baking soda to the machine's rinse cycle to remove detergent completely from clothes.
- **Drying Clothes** - In summer months try to use a clothesline. I know it is hard to imagine but it will save money and teach your family about the old days. After your clothes are dry you can put them in the dryer for a couple of minutes to soften them up.
- **Fabric Softener** - Add a few drops of Purification, Lavender, Joy or other oil on a wet rag and place in the dryer or mist from a spray bottle directly into the dryer.

POLISHING

- **Brass, Copper, Bronze and Aluminum** - To remove tarnish, rub metal with sliced lemons. For tough jobs, sprinkle baking soda on the lemon, then rub. Polish metal, clean copper, bronze and brass with a paste of white vinegar and salt; rub metal, then rinse and dry.
- **Sterling Silver** - Put a sheet of aluminum foil into a plastic or glass bowl. Sprinkle the foil with salt and baking soda, and then fill the bowl with warm water. Just soak your silver in the bowl and the tarnish will migrate to the aluminum foil. Finally, rinse, dry, and buff your silver with a soft cloth or make a paste of baking soda and water, put some on a clean, soft rag, and polish. Rinse and polish dry.
- **Furniture Polish** - Use 1 tsp. olive oil per ½ cup vinegar. It will extract dirt and moisturize and protect wood. Tips: To remove water spots, rub well with home-made toothpaste. To remove scratches, use 1 part lemon juice and 1 part olive oil; rub with a soft cloth.

FLOORS AND CARPETS

- **Linoleum, Tile, Brick or Stone** - 1 cup vinegar or Borax in 1 gal. of warm water or 1/4 cup baking soda with 1 Tbsp of liquid soap, 1/4 cup vinegar and 2 gal. hot water. Put the soda in the bucket first and add the liquid ingredients. CAUTION: Do not use this formula on waxed floors! For an extra polish, combine 6 Tbsp of cornstarch per cup of water in a bucket.

- **Wood and Other Types of Floors** - Vinegar is a natural disinfectant, and it pulls dirt from wood. I use 1 cup distilled white vinegar per pail of hot water to clean my wood floors (1/2 cup vinegar to 1 gal. water); The smell disappears immediately. Do NOT use on wood finished with polyurethane.
- **Carpet Spills** - when you have a current spill on a carpet, don't blot dry; just pour a large amount of morton salt directly on the spill and let stand until dry. Then scoop up and vacuum. Thanks, Marcie Decker.
- **Carpet** - Sprinkle baking soda over the surface of the carpet and let it stand for 15 to 30 minutes before vacuuming. This will soak up spills and eliminate odors.
- **Vacuum** – Use Thieves Spray on vacuum filters. It makes great clean air.

PEST CONTROL

- **Insecticide** - dust mites, fleas, ticks, ants, spiders, etc. Essential oils and oil blends such as citronella, lavender, lemon, peppermint, lemongrass, cypress, eucalyptus globulus, cinnamon, thyme, basil, Thieves, and Purification effectively repel many types of insects, including mites, lice, and fleas. Peppermint placed on entryways prevents ants from entering.
- **Ants**-Mix sugar or cinnamon with baking soda 50/50, sprinkle where you need it.
- **Bug Repellent** - To make an insect repellent use 5 drops each of palo santos, eucalyptus and citronella in a 2 oz. (50 ml) spritzer with either water or olive oil.
- **Bug Bite Ointment** - Mix 2 oz. water and 10 drops of each/or separate olive oil, coconut oil, or YLEO V-6 oil. Add equal parts of peppermint, lavender, patchouli, lemongrass, or any oil you prefer and put on location.
- **Moth Repellent** - If you need moth repellent for your linens and woolens, avoid toxic commercial mothballs made of naphthalene. Essential oils such as lavender, lemongrass, Canadian red cedar, or rosemary can just as effectively repel moths and other insects. You can make a sachet by placing several drops of essential oil on a cotton ball. Wrap and tie this in a small handkerchief or square of cotton. Hang this cloth in storage areas or add it to your chest of linens. Refresh as often as necessary.

WHAT DO ESSENTIAL OILS DO FOR YOU WHEN THEY ARE DIFFUSED?

When essential oils are diffused, the molecules are broken up into micro-fine mist particles. These mist particles stay suspended in the air for long periods of time. Not only does this reduce bacteria, mold, and odors in the air, but these micro-mist particles also benefit those who inhale them. Diffused oils do more than mask odors; they actually alter the structure of the molecules that create odors - rendering them harmless! They also increase the available oxygen in the room and produce negative ions. Research at Webber State University shows that diffusing essential oils destroys airborne microorganisms. Diffusing is so effective that many hospitals in England and France diffuse essential oils daily to keep incidences of drug-resistant bacteria low and to keep the air free from microorganisms.

MISCELLANEOUS INFORMATION

- **Vampire Electricity** - Many appliances use electricity - up to 40% of the full power - when you are not using them. Using the Smart Plug (seen on Oprah) can save you money. Visit www.amazon.com and type in "Smart-Strip."
- **Cleaning Fruits and Vegetables** - I have heard that using lemon, peroxide, or vinegar as a veggie wash cleans off pesticides and herbicides. This is one of the furthest things from the truth! Whether the crop was sprayed as a seedling or a plant; it affects the skin as well as the inside of the plant. See ewg.org/node/22100 for "dirty dozen" also "Future of Food" video at livinganointed.com/links.html. Visit www.organicbythecase.com for organic food any time of the year.
- **Sticky Residues** - Lemon or citrus oils take gum, labels, or any type of glue from bottles.
- Sleepwear - Lavender and roman chamomile is especially fragrant and relaxing.

Research also shows that cold-air diffusing certain oils may:

1. Reduce bacteria, fungus, mold, and unpleasant odors.
2. Relax the mind and body, relieve tension, and clear the mind.
3. Help with weight management.
4. Improve concentration, alertness, and mental clarity.
5. Purify the air and neutralize mildew, cigarette smoke, etc.
6. Improve your home, work, or study environment.
7. Help you experience the calming and emotionally balancing effects of certain essential oils.

What to do with Toxic Products?

First, when you find a product you like, call the company and see if they have coupons. If you have toxic products at home, you can return them to the store, and you don't even need a receipt! I got $150.00 back! Gather all of the toxic products, separate them by store then make sure they haven't expired. Then gather all of the products for each store and take back all of the products from one store at a time, i.e get all Kroger's items and take back to get your store credit. You are only allowed to take back goods to a store with no receipt 1-2 times, so it's best to do all at one time. Bring this book, show warning labels, etc.

Most companies have a satisfaction guarantee, call them and give your 2cents (hopefully it will make a difference) and they will send your money back.

Demand that the government require companies to disclose product ingredients and replace toxic chemicals with safer alternatives. Contact your congressional representative and ask them to support legislation that would require companies to disclose their product ingredients completely. Also ask them to support chemical policy reform.

For more information go to: http://database.healthandenvironment.org/
www.louisvillecharter.org/ • http://www.watoxics.org/homes-and-gardens/fastfacts/fastfacts-cleaning

Easy Homemade Recommendations

Personal Care Products

Today, most skin and hair care products contain harmful petrochemicals that cause allergic reactions and skin and scalp irritations. Mineral oils and sodium lauryl sulfate dehydrate the skin and cause allergies, dandruff, and scalp rashes. Chemical molecules plug the pores of the skin, causing loss of oxygen and irritation.

On the other hand, essential oil molecules are absorbed into the derma and subderma skin cells to oxygenate, regenerate, and re-hydrate the cells. Young Living skin care products, which are free of petrochemicals and animal products, are formulated with all-natural ingredients. Essential oils are the perfect products for maintaining beautiful, healthy skin.

How To Stay Regular

Many folks use metamucil on a regular basises. It would be a better chose to use one of the following examples. Put the following into a blender: one 8oz glass of water, 1 Tbs. of olive oil, 2 Tbs. of flax seed oil, and the juice of one lemon. Grate 1/2 of the lemon's rind and a piece of fresh ginger root 1 inch by 1 inch and add. Blend for 1 min. Drink on an empty stomach. Or use 1tsp. of celtic sea salt in 12-16oz of warm water day or night.

Mouthwash

Mix 4-6 drops of Thieves and 3-4 drops of peppermint in 16 oz. of water. Use twice a day minimum, shake, gargle, then swallow. Use these oils as a base and change it up as you need for kids such as adding in some orange maybe a little less Thieves etc. For oral hygiene or dental issues add extra clove, wintergreen, & thyme oil.

Toothpaste

Mix 2 drops of Thieves and 2 drops of peppermint in a small jar (the size of a jelly jar). Fill half way with baking soda, put lid on, and shake vigorously. If you see any clumps, just smush with your finger or a spoon, then fill up with more baking soda. Get your toothbrush wet and dip in the jar and brush. YLEO has Thieves toothpaste and 4 kinds to choose from. See how to videos at LivingAnointed.com

Deodorants

Young Living deodorant is the best, they have two to choose from. It contains essential oils that help clean out your lymphatic system and remove toxins.

Foot Deodorant

Lavender Deodorant on feet and wipe off excess. Helps neutralize odors and makes skin silky, smooth and fresh.

Genital Deodorant

Apple Cider Vinegar-Lavender Deodorant is excellent for cleansing the body, neutralizing odors and keeping the natural bacteria in balance. Use as needed as a spray or douche. No rinsing necessary.

Hair Rinse

Raw apple cider vinegar removes shampoo and chemical residue while adding softness and shine. The high acid content plus the enzymes kill bacteria that can cause such problems as itching scalp and dandruff. Mix 1/3 cup apple cider vinegar and 4 cups of warm water. Shampoo and rinse hair, squeezing out excess water, then pour apple cider mixture over your hair and rub into your scalp. Leave on at least one minute, then rinse.

Baby / Body Wipes

Making your own baby wipes will save your baby's health and your money. You can be assured there are no harsh or drying chemicals on anyone's skin. Use an empty wipe container.

1. Flatten and cut a roll of paper towels in half. Remove the inner cardboard core.
2. Combine the YLEO liquid soap with 1 cup of water and pour it into the container.
3. Place the paper towel in container and turn it around,
4. If there are still any dry spots add 1/4 cup of water.
5. Pull the towel from the center of the roll.
6. Wipes are now ready to use. You can perfect your own recipe.

Body Wipes Recipe

2 Tbsp castile soap i.e., Dr. Woods, Kirks, Dr. Bronners
2 Tbsp olive oil, 2 drops tea tree oil, 1 drop of Lavender
2 cups water
You can add 1/4 cup aloe vera gel. Now, mix well in your wipes box

Sunscreen

We need sun rays; it is the best source of Vitamin D. I mix coconut oil and Lavendar and Frankinsence oil together. Lavendar protects the skin from burning as well as if someone is burned. The A.R.T Skincare system is a great anti-aging Peptide complex to restore and protect skin. The most chemical free sunscreen I have found is Dr. Mercola Natural Sunscreen for adults and children at www.mercola.com..

Antibiotic Ointment

Use Young Living Animal Scents Ointment and/or Melrose oil right to open wound.

Vegetable Wash

Pesticide residues on fruit and vegetables can not be just washed off. Apple cider vinegar, Lemon Oil, Thieves Cleaner and Baking Soda. I put a little baking soda in my hand, then spray it with Thieves Cleaner, then with my hands scrub the fruits and veggies.

Mosquitoes

To prevent mosquitoe bites use citronella, lavender, or/and lemongrass. Mix with YLEO V6 or coconut oil and rub on. For a great bite pain reliever use a mixture of patchouli, peppermint and lavender. FYI, when your pH is balanced the mosquitoes won't bug you!

Motion Sickness

Mix patchouli, peppermint and lavender and rub on the mastoid (bone just behind the ear) and bellybutton and then breathe in. If you do this 30 minutes before a trip you will be able to read, etc... and not get sick.

Organic Pest Control

We can repel bugs naturally. Purchase a glass spray bottle and fill it with pure water and add YLEO to spray around the home inside/out, plants, pets, car, etc. (I recommend 10 drops to 2 oz water.) If you are bitten/stung by red ants, wasps or bees, Purification & Lavender Oil will neutralize the venom immediately and reduce the swelling.

The following is a list of specific oils to eliminate bugs:
Ants, Caterpillars, Plant Lice, Spiders — Peppermint and Spearmint
Aphids, Lice, Moths — Cedarwood, Hyssop, Peppermint, Spearmint, Lavender
Beetles — Peppermint and Thyme
Fleas — Peppermint, Lemongrass, Spearmint, Lavender
Flies — Lavender, Peppermint, Rosemary, Sage
Gnats — Patchouli, Spearmint
Mosquitoes — Lavender, Lemongrass
Slugs, Snails — Cedarwood, Hyssop, Pine, Patchouli
Ticks — Lavender, Lemongrass, Sage, Thyme

Other Companies I like
- Organic By The Case (USA wide) www.organicbythecase.com
- Zcoil Shoes www.zcoil.com is the best shoe you will ever wear. They have shoes for all ages and sizes. Let them know I sent you, they have a referral program.

Must have Appliances:
- **Cuisinart Griddler**- a countertop grill. Khols.com or bedbathandbeyond.com.
- **Juicer** - there are many different kinds
- **Vita-Mix** - a high-performance whole food blender that is famous for its durability, dependability and amazing warranty. To purchase go to LivingAnointed.com or call Vita Mix at 800-848-2649. For (savings of $25 U.S.) use code *06-003176*
- **Glass Nebulizer Essential Oil Diffuser** - Check out s at LivingAnointed.com.
- **Diffuser Necklaces** - The best I have seen are at www.personaldiffusers.com.

Good Products to Purchase
- Stoneyfield Farm Organic: www.stoneyfield.com
- Lifeway Kefir: www.lifeway.net
- Chocolate Bars by Raw Indulgence: www.glutensmart.com
- CocoaCassava: chocolate bars: www.cocoacassava.com
- Chocolate, mints or gum- www.naturessunshine.com (Ruth Dec 810-733-0701)
- Spry gum and mints
- Applegate Farms meats
- Deitz and Watson Deli Meat (No MSG) www.dietzandwatson.com
- Food for Life: Ezekiel 4:9 Bread & Tortillas; www.foodforlife.com
- Kashi: www.kashi.com
- Sunview Raisins
- Kettle Brand Plain Chips (some have "flavors", which is MSG)
- Newman's Own (anything to do with Paul Newman's brand is good)
- Celtic Salt or Pink Himalayan Salt
- Green Pastures- Organic Coconut Oil and Ghee greenpastures.org
- Wholesome Sweeteners Organic Agave Nectar: www.amazon.com
- Young Living (YL) NingXia Wolfberries and NingXia Red: LivingAnointed.com
- Cloth Diapers: www.diapersafari.com
- Thermal, leak proof straw bottle, sippy cup & food jar: www.thermos.com
- Organic Toddler baby formula: www.naturesone.com/dairy.php
- Seventh Generation: www.seventhgeneration.com
- Farm Boy Tortilla Chips with a flavor and no MSG: www.farmboyflapjacks.com

Vitacost.com- you can purchase the following: Dr. Christophers Liq. Cayenne, Carlson Liq. Vit D, Nutiva Coconut Oil, Nutivia Hemp Hearts/powder, Dr. woods soap and Spry Gum or mints. Good prices-but not everything on vitacost is straight.

Extra Curricular Activities... Sex

Are you missing something? Do you have a loss of desire for intimacy, or do you just need help with lubrication? Young Livings Essential oils can help mentally, physically and emotionally!

Engaging in "Extra Curricular Activities" is an important part of married life. It is meant to be enjoyed, reproduce life, and strengthen the emotional bond between partners. It is a concern for both involved if one does not have sexual desires (low libido) or is experiencing any type of physical issues that may hinder his or her performance. Low libido is not just a physical issue. Our minds are very powerful. Low self-esteem, insecurity regarding sexual ability or physical appearances can weaken the ego and hinder one's desire for intimacy. Even more tragic is when our sexuality has been shaped by others. A lack of loving support and compassion from a partner when dealing with any of the above issue can be devastating. But imagine the effects on someone who has never experienced any traumatic sexual experience. Here's the good news, it can be over come. There is hope! Please read the emotional response section of the Young Living Desk refference to see what oils work the best.

The only oils I suggest for vaginal use are the Young Living Essential Oils. In fact, all my oil suggestions are the use of Young Living Essential Oils. Read on, and have fun but use good judgment on what oils to use and how much. I have been told that there are actual health benefits associated with Extra Curricular Activities such as, muscle toning, immunity, stress, cardiovascular strength, and most of all it promotes emotional bonding. It really can bring one closer to their partner, by becoming relaxed, happy and tension free.

First, if you don't have a desire for sex, your hormones need to be checked whether you are female or male. Next, review your diet, your water intake, most likely a nutritional cleanse and fast are at hand (Chapter 3). Most women have had great success with taking YL PD 80/20 and YL Progessence Plus Serum. Men, it is amazing how many husbands are happier just from the YL Progessence Plus! Also, the Men's YL Prostate Health capsules, YL NingXia Red drink and the Prostrate Rectal application recipe* (located at the end of this chapter) are packed with the oil combination needed to maintain good health. Some guys call the Prostrate Rectal procedure their 6 month lube and tune.

No Testimonies Here

Not from personal experience but, after I had a hysterectomy (before I knew better) I needed to use a lubricant. This was prior to learning about toxic chemicals in our everyday products. The lubricant never really seemed to work. The two main ingredients in personal lubricants such as KY Jelly are propylene glycol and polyethylene glycol. Those ingredients will dry the vaginal canal. I kept using the lubricant, because of the drying effect of the lubricant, this caused an addiction to the lubricant. Because of the toxic lubricants I developed chronic bladder and yeast infections. (as if I didn't have enough problems.)

Now for the good stuff

Essential oils can enhance the sexual experience in several ways. The scent of the oil will create the 'mood' by stimulating our olfactory nerves. The sense of smell is directly linked to areas of the brain that regulate the release of hormones. These hormones affect the limbic part of the brain that triggers one's emotions promoting, attraction and arousal for both women and men. The molecules of oils are so small that they pass the blood brain barrier and get right into the bloodstream within 3 seconds to 20 minutes, circulating throughout the whole body.

Lubricants

The best sexual lubricant is natural vaginal secretion. The next best is saliva, unless you have a known oral or gum disease. When more is needed, use coconut oil or YL V6.

Essential Oils known for their aphrodisiac properties

You can use the oils listed below in a diffuser, they can be used on your body and they can also be used on linens. Of course the key here is to use good judgment.

- **Massage** - body, hand, foot etc. add a few drops of YLEO to a 'base' oil, such as coconut oil, YLEO V6 or almond oil. NOTE: Do not use baby or mineral oil or regular lotions with YLEO, you will have a undesirable reaction mixing YLEO with petroleum based products.
- **On body** - old fashion real vanilla extract is great, YL Stress away, YL Tangerine or YL Peppermint oil, Ortho Ease Massage oil or any oil you like to smell or taste. Use anywhere on body you want to nibble or naw at.
- **Vaginal** - using a lubricant type mentioned from above, mix your favorite YLEO in it, YLEO Ortho Ease Massage oil or ClaraDerm Spray as needed.
- **Bath** - 5-10 drops in bath water like YL Lavender, YL Fennel, i.e., again any oil you like the smell of and that relaxes you.
- **Diffuse** - Choose any scent you like: YL Cinnamon bark, YL Christmas spirit, YL Fennel, YL Anise, YL Citrus oils especially YL Tangerine. Ylang Ylang is very stimulating, however if you dislike the smell use it on the bottom of your feet.
- **Spritz** - on linen, around the room and yourself - In a 2 oz bottle spray bottle, fill with pure water, add 5 drops of the oil you both like.

Additional YLEO recommendations you can use for arousing effects:

Grapefruit, Orange, Tangerine or any citrus oils refreshes and energizes the senses. Citrus Oils have a photosensitivity so don't go directly into the sunlight after you applied topically.

Cedarwood - with a woody aroma, it is reassuring and infuses warmth into the atmosphere.

Clary Sage - acts as a tonic for the female reproduction system and boosts sexual confidence.

Rose - is almost synonymous with love and romance. It's fresh, floral scent is a powerful aphrodisiac.

Patchouli - is good for treating sexual problems such as impotency, loss of libido, lack of interest, erectile problems, frigidity etc. Patchouli also acts as an aphrodisiac.

Ylang Ylang - considered one of the most powerful aphrodisiacs. Ylang Ylang increases libido and attraction between lovers. It energizes, intensifies eroticism and is good for sexual experimentation.

Ginger - has a warm and cozy aroma that creates a cozy atmosphere for couples making lovemaking last longer.

Nutmeg - helps to overcome frigidity.

Cinnamon Bark - taste and smell is invigorating. Use with caution, it is a hot oil. Start out with 1 drop at a time.

Peppermint - taste, smell and feels invigorating. Use with caution, it is a hot oil. Start out with 1 drop at a time.

Jasmine - lifts the mood and adds to the energy levels. Traditionally, it is used to combat frigidity, impotence and premature ejaculation, thanks to its powerful erogenous effect.

Lavender - increases blood flow to genitals and enhances female sensitivity.

Sandalwood - works wonders for men. The sweet, woody and exotic scent enhances physical sensuality and makes lovers more sexually-liberated. Considered a sexual restorative, it induces a state of calmness and serenity and relieves nervous tension.

Black Pepper and Sandalwood - mixing these oils can give a boost to a man's vigor.

Other great blends- Sensation, Valor and Joy.

*Prostrate Blend Recipe - YL Protec or Organic coconut oil, 4 ounce bottle with dropper, Young Living Essential oils: Mister, EndoFlex, Thyme, Wintergreen, Frankincense, Myrrh, Sage, Cypress, Juniper, Helichrysum, Balsam Fir.

Add 15 drops of each of the listed oils into a 4" glass eye droper bottle, fill the bottle with the Protec or olive oil, or YLEO V6. Shake the bottle well. Before going to sleep, while lying down insert the 4" glass eye droper rectally with one full dropper, as far up the rectum as possible. Continue this procedure every night for a total of 6 nights and schedule it again in 6 months. Or in severe situations after 6 nights use the oil every other night until for 2 weeks then re-address situation. Refer to prostate testimonies at LivingAnointed.com.

Please send your 'clean' testimonial so we can share more ideas.

Everything You Wanted To Know About Essential Oils

God's Intelligence in Oils

The beauty of having the oils as medicine is that they don't have negative side effects like synthetic drugs and chemicals of modern pharmacology. "…The leaf thereof shall be your medicine." Ezekiel 47:12. The tinctures of iodine, merthiolate, mercurochrome, and other antiseptics may be effective in killing organisms that invade open wounds, but they are toxic and destructive to human tissue and retard healing as well. Please look into reading Dr. David Stewart's book, "Healing Oils of the Bible".

The Worlds Leader in Essential Oils

D. Gary Young's commitment to understanding the remarkable therapeutic power of plants has resulted in the world's largest line of therapeutic grade essential oils and blends. Gary has traveled the globe discovering how to best support both physical health and emotional wellness. His discoveries have helped hundreds of thousands of people experience the benefits of natural healing and have led to the creation of the world's largest and foremost authority on essential oils sciences: Young Living Essential Oils.

Gary Young established the term "therapeutic-grade," now known as Young Living Therapeutic Grade™ (YLTG), as a guarantee that Young Living will only sell 100% pure, natural, uncut oils that maintain the vital therapeutic potency.

As Gary traveled the world studying the distillation of pure essential oils, he saw wide discrepancies in quality and learned that in order to ensure purity and potency, expert, rigorous analysis of finished oils was critical.

Today, using gas chromatography (GC) and mass spectrometry (MS) analysis, the phytochemical profile of every batch of Young Living essential oils is measured to evaluate each specific plant compound. Certain plant compounds must meet or exceed specific levels to ensure the oil is natural, pure, and therapeutic-grade. Only then does Young Living guarantee the oil will provide the desired results and label it Young Living Therapeutic Grade™ (YLTG).

The six Young Living farms and distilleries—located in Mona, Utah, U.S.; St. Maries, Idaho, U.S.; Simiane-la-Rotonde, France; Guayaquil, Ecuador; Salalah, Oman; and Lima, Peru- allow Young Living Essential Oils to maintain its position as the world's leading grower, distiller, and provider of pure, potent essential oils.

On Young Living farms, the cultivation, harvesting, and distillation processes of each batch of essential oils are carefully controlled. Extensive laboratory testing and independent audits are conducted to ensure Young Living's quality exceeds industry standards. Experimentation performed on Young Living farms helps guarantee the consistent quality of YLTG, and allows for increased research and development opportunities.

It is this hands-on experience of growing, distilling, sourcing, and testing essential oils that led to the development of the Seed to Seal™ process. This method, exclusive to Young Living Essential Oils, ensures that each Young Living essential oil product delivers the quality results customers have come to expect.

Mankind's First Medicine

For many centuries essential oils and other aromatics were used for religious rituals, treatment of illness, and other physical and spiritual needs. Records dating back to 450 BC describe the use of balsamic substances with aromatic properties for religious rituals and medical applications. Ancient writings tell of scented barks, resins, spices, aromatic vinegars, wines, and beers that were used in rituals, temples, astrology, embalming, and medicine.

The Egyptians were masters in using essential oils and other aromatics in the embalming process. Historical records describe how one of the founders of "pharaonic" medicine was the architect Imhotep, who was the Grand Vizier of King Djoser (2780 - 2720 BC). Imhotep is often given credit for ushering in the use of oils, herbs, and aromatic plants for medicinal purposes. Many hieroglyphics on the walls of Egyptian temples depict the blending of oils and describe hundreds of oil recipes.

An ancient papyrus, found in the Temple of Edfu, contains medicinal formulas and perfume recipes used by alchemists and high priests in blending aromatic substances for rituals. The Egyptians may have been the first to discover the potential of fragrance. They created various aromatic blends for both personal use and ceremonies performed in the temples and pyramids.

Well before the time of Christ, the ancient Egyptians collected essential oils and placed them in alabaster vessels. These vessels were specially carved and shaped for housing scented oils. In 1922, when King Tut's tomb was opened, some 50 alabaster jars designed to hold 350 liters of oil were discovered. Tomb robbers had stolen nearly all of the precious oil, leaving the jars behind. Some of them still contained oil traces.

In 1817, the Ebers Papyrus, a medical scroll over 870 feet long, was discovered. Dating back to 1500 BC, the scroll included over 800 different herbal prescriptions and remedies. Other scrolls describe a high success rate in treating 81 different diseases. Many of the remedies contained myrrh and honey. Myrrh is still recognized for its ability to help with infections of the skin and throat and to regenerate skin tissue. Myrrh was used for embalming because of its effectiveness in preventing bacterial growth.

The physicians of Ionia, Attica, and Crete (ancient civilizations based in the Mediterranean Sea) came to the cities of the Nile to increase their knowledge. Hippocrates (460-377 BC), whom the Greeks dubbed (with perhaps some exaggeration) "The Father of Medicine" founded and taught at the school of Cos. The Romans purified their temples, and political buildings by **diffusing essential oils.** They also used aromatics in their steam baths to both invigorate the flesh, and ward off disease.

What Is an Essential Oil?

Essential oils are aromatic volatile liquids distilled from plants, shrubs, flowers, trees, roots, bushes, and seeds. The chemistry of essential oils is very complex: each one may consist of hundreds of different and unique chemical compounds. Moreover, essential oils are highly concentrated and far more potent than dried herbs. The distillation process is what makes essential oils so concentrated. It often requires an entire plant (or more) to produce a single drop of distilled essential oil. Essential oils contain oxygenating molecules, which transport the nutrients to the cells of the body. Without oxygen, nutrients cannot be assimilated, leaving us nutritionally depleted.

Essential oils are also different from vegetable oils such as corn oil, peanut oil, and olive oil. They are not greasy and do not clog the pores like many vegetable oils. Vegetable oils can become oxidized, and rancid over time and are not antibacterial. Most essential oils, on the other hand, cannot go rancid and are powerful antimicrobials. Pressed oils and essential oils that are high in plant waxes (such as patchouli), if not distilled properly, could go rancid over time, particularly if exposed to heat for extended periods of time.

Essential oils are substances that definitely deserve the respect of proper education. Users need to be fully versed in the chemistry and safety of the oils. However, this knowledge is not being taught at universities in the United States. There is a disturbing lack of institutional information, knowledge, and training on essential oils and the scientific approach to aromatherapy. Only in the Middle East, the Orient, and Europe, (with their far longer history of using natural products and botanical extracts) can one obtain adequate instruction on the chemistry and therapy of essential oils.

How Do Essential Oils Work?

Essential oils are not simple substances. The limbic system is the processing center for reason, emotion, and smell. Each essential oil contains as many as 100 chemical components, which together exert a strong effect on the whole person. Depending on which component is predominating in an oil, the oil acts differently. For example, some oils are relaxing, some soothe you, some relieve pain, etc. Then there are oils, such as lemon and lavender, which adapt to what your body needs. These are called "adaptogenic". The mechanism in which these essential oils act on us is not very well understood. What is understood, however is that they affect our mind and emotions. They leave no harmful residues. They enter into the body either by absorption or inhalation.

A fragrance company in Japan conducted studies to determine the effects of smell on people. They pumped different fragrances into an area where a number of keyboard entry operators were stationed and monitored the number of mistakes made. The results are as follows:

- When exposed to lavender oil fragrance (a relaxant), typing errors dropped 20%.
- When exposed to jasmine (an uplifting fragrance), the errors dropped 33%.
- When exposed to lemon (a sharp, refreshing stimulant), the mistakes fell by 54%!

An essential oil can have widely different actions depending on its chemistry. Some essential oil company's basil don't have any methyl chavicol. Where basil high in methyl chavicol is more anti-inflammatory and anti- spasmotic. A third type, basil high in eugenol, has both anti-inflammatory and antiseptic effects.

Essential oils can be distilled or extracted in different ways that have dramatic effects on their chemistry and medicinal action. Oils derived from a second or third distillation of the same plant material, are obviously not going to be as potent as oils extracted during the first distillation. Oils that are subjected to high heat and pressure have a distinctly simpler and inferior profile of chemical constituents as well. Excessive heat and temperature fractures and breaks down many of the delicate aromatic compounds within the oil, some of which are responsible for its therapeutic action. Oils that are steam distilled are far different from those that are solvent extracted.

The Benefits Of Young Living Therapeutic Grade Essential Oils

1. Essential oils are so small in molecular size they can penetrate the skin.
2. Essential oils are lipid soluble and are capable of penetrating cell walls, even those hardened because of oxygen deficiency. Essential oils can affect every cell of the body within 20 minutes and are metabolized like other nutrients.
3. Essential oils contain oxygen molecules, which help transport nutrients to cells. Because nutritional deficiency is an oxygen deficiency, disease begins when cells lack oxygen for proper nutrient assimilation. By providing oxygen, essential oils work to stimulate the immune system.
4. Essential oils are powerful antioxidants that create an unfriendly environment for free radicals. They work as free-radical scavengers, prevent cell mutation, prevent fungus, and prevent cellular oxidation.
5. Essential oils have been shown to destroy bacteria and viruses while simultaneously restoring physiological balance to the body.
6. Essential oils may detoxify cells and blood in the body.
7. Essential oils containing sesquiterpenes have the ability to pass through the blood-brain barrier.
8. Essential oils are aromatic and when diffused may provide air purification by:
    a. Removing metallic particles and toxins from the air.
    b. Increasing atmospheric oxygen.
    c. Increasing ozone and negative ions in the air, which inhibit bacterial growth.
    d. Eliminating odors from mold, cigarettes, and animals.
9. Essential oils promote physical, emotional, and spiritual well being.
10. Essential oils have a bioelectrical frequency that is several times greater than the frequency of herbs, food and even the human body.

11. Clinical research has shown that essential oils can quickly raise the frequency of the human body, restoring it to its normal, healthy level. Electrical frequencies range from 52 MHz to 320 MHz. See livinganointed.com/healing/frequencies.

12. All essential oils containing sesquiterpenes are known to give oxygen to cells.

13. Increased secretions of endorphins, antibodies, serotonin and hormones.

15. Increased production of ATP (energy fuel used by cells).

18. Increased histamine release, which speeds up the healing process.

19. Increased conversion of amino acids and proteins.

20. Help in promotion of secretion and receptivity of human growth hormone (HGH).

Before You Start Using Essential Oils, Know These Basic Guidelines for Safe Use

Purchase your own copy of "Essential Oil Desk Reference Book" @ ylwisdom.com

1. **Always do a skin test before applying a new oil to the skin.** Each person's body is different, so apply oils to a small area first. Apply oils one at a time. When layering oils that are new to you, allow a few minutes for the body to respond before applying a second oil. NOTE: If your body pH balance is low (means your body is very acidic), you could have a negative reaction to the oils. See pH Balance and Acidosis document. You can drink 1tsp. of baking soda in 8 oz. of water or put fresh squeezed lemon in your water or 5 drops of YLEO lemon oil.

2. Exercise caution when applying essential oils to skin that has been exposed to **any petrochemical** such as aluminum, sodium laurel sulfate, propylene glycol, lead acetate, vaseline, mineral oil, baby oil or other synthetic chemicals (see Toxic Chemical List). These are often found in cosmetics, toothpaste, mouthwash, deodorants, and skin and personal care products, soaps, perms, hair colors or dyes, hair sprays, gels and cleansers. Some chemicals, (especially petroleum-based chemicals), can penetrate and remain in the skin and fatty tissues for days or even weeks after use. Essential oils may react with such chemicals and cause skin irritation, nausea, headaches, or other uncomfortable effects.

3. Essential oils can also react with toxins built up in the body from chemicals in food, water, and the work environment. If you experience a reaction to essential oils, it may be wise to temporarily discontinue their use and start an internal cleansing program before resuming regular use.

4. Always keep a bottle of pure YL V-6 Vegetable Mixing Oil, olive or coconut oil (base oil) handy when using essential oils. Use a pure oil to dilute essential oils if they cause discomfort or skin irritation. If skin irritation persist, discontinue using the oil on that location and apply the oils on the bottoms of the feet.

5. Always drink half your body weight in ounces of pure water to flush out toxins.

6. Keep bottles of essential oils tightly closed and store in a cool location away from light heat. If stored properly, they will maintain their potency for years.

7. Keep essential oils out of reach of children. Treat them as any product for therapeutic use. If a child or infant swallows an essential oil, administer a mixture of milk, cream, yogurt, or safe, oil-soluble liquid.

8. Essential oils rich in menthol (such as peppermint) should not be used on the throat or neck area of children under 30 months of age.

9. Angelica, bergamot, grapefruit, lemon, tangerine, and other citrus oils are photosensitive, and may cause a rash or dark pigmentation on skin exposed to direct sunlight or UV rays within 3-4 days after application. Drinking the citrus oils, however, is fine.

10. Keep essential oils well away from the eye area and never put them directly into ears. **Do not handle contact lenses or rub eyes with essential oils on your fingers.** Even in minimal amounts, oils with high phenol content, such as Oregano, Cinnamon Bark, thyme, Clove, Lemongrass, and Bergamot, may damage contacts and will irritate eyes. Immediate dilution is strongly recommended if skin becomes painfully irritated or if oil accidentally gets into eyes. Flushing the area with coconut, olive, or V6 oil will minimize discomfort almost immediately. Do NOT flush with water! Essential oils are oil-soluble, not water-soluble.

11. Pregnant women should consult a professional when starting a health program.

12. Epileptics and those with high blood pressure should consult their health care professional before using essential oils. Please see the Essential Oil Desk Reference.

14. People with allergies should test a small amount of oil on an area of sensitive skin, such as the inside of the upper arm, then wait for 30 minutes before applying the oil on other areas. The bottom of the feet is one of the safest places to start.

15. Before taking GRAS (Generally Regarded As Safe, listed in Appendix B) essential oils internally, test your reactions by diluting one drop of essential oil in 1 tsp. of an oil soluble liquid like agave, olive oil, or rice milk.

16. Do not add undiluted essential oils directly to bath water. Using Epsom salts or a bath gel base for oils applied to your bath is an excellent way to disperse the oils into the bath water. When essential oils are put directly into bath water without a dispersing agent, they can cause serious discomfort on sensitive skin because the essential oils float, (undiluted), on top of the water.

17. Keep essential oils away from open flames, sparks, or electricity. Some essential oils, including orange, fir, pine, and peppermint are potentially flammable.

18. Do not mix oil blends. Someone who understands the chemical constituents of each oil, and which oils blend well, has specially formulated commercially available blends. The chemical properties of the oils can be altered when mixed improperly, resulting in some undesirable reactions.

Essential Oils Application

TOPICAL APPLICATIONS

1. **Direct Application** - Apply the oils directly on the area of concern using one to six drops of oil. More oil is not necessarily better since a large amount of oil can trigger a detoxification of the surrounding tissue and blood. Such a quick detoxification can be somewhat uncomfortable. Layering individual oils is preferred over mixing your own blends. Layering refers to the process of applying one oil, rubbing it in, and then applying another oil. There is no need to wait more than a couple of seconds between each oil as absorption occurs quite rapidly. If dilution is necessary, the Base Oil may be applied on top. This technique is not only useful in physical healing, but also when doing emotional clearing.

2. **Vita Flex Therapy** was developed by Stanley Burroughs after more than fifty years of research and application. Vita Flex Therapy is a simple method of applying oils to contact points (or nerve endings) in the feet or hands. A series of hand rotation movements at those control points create a vibration healing energy that carries the oils along the neuroelectrical pathways. The oils help increase the frequency of this healing energy. They serve to either help remove any blockage along the pathways, or travel the length of the pathway to benefit the particular organ.

3. **Raindrop Technique** was developed by Gary Young and is a simple application of dropping certain oils like drops of rain from about six inches above the body along the entire length of the spine. It is a tremendous boost to the immune system as it releases toxins and kills viruses and bacteria that have accumulated along the spine.

4. **Auricular Therapy** - A method of applying the oils to the rim of the ears. This technique works extremely well for emotional clearing. Some physical benefits can also be obtained from this technique.

5. **Perfumes or Cologne** - Wearing the oils as a perfume or cologne can provide wonderful emotional and physical support.

INTERNALLY

1. The FDA has approved some essential oils for internal use and given them the designation of **GRAS** (Generally Regarded As Safe for internal consumption).

2. **Taking Orally** - YLEO are very effective when taken internally. Essential oils should always be diluted in agave nectar, V6 oil, coconut oil, olive oil or rice milk. Read specific oil for dilution amounts.

3. **Vaginal Retention** - Used for systemic health problems such as candida or vaginitis. Vaginal retention is one of the best ways for the body to absorb essential oils. Mix 20 to30 drops of essential oil in 2 Tbsp. of carrier oil. Apply this mixture to a tampon (for internal infection) or sanitary pad (for external lesions). Insert and retain for 8 hours or overnight. Use tampons made with organic cotton.
4. **Rectal Retention** - Enemas are the most efficient way to deliver essential oils to the urinary tract and reproductive organs. Always use a sterile syringe. Mix 15 to 20 drops of essential oil in a Tbsp. of carrier oil. Place the mixture in a small syringe and inject into the rectum. Retain the mixture through the night (or longer for best results).

DO NOT attempt to do this with any store bought essential oil unless it says for internal or dietary use. Even those found at a health food store may not be pure enough!

COMPRESSES

1. **Massage** - Apply a hot wet towel under a dry towel on top of an already massaged area. The moist heat will force the oils deeper into the tissues of the body.

INHALATIONS

1. **Directly Inhale** - Place 2 or more drops in the palm of your left hand, and rub clockwise with the flat palm of your right hand. Cup your hands together over the nose and mouth and inhale deeply. (Do not touch your eyes!)
2. **Diffuse** - The easiest and simplest way of putting the oils into the air for inhalation is to use an aromatic mist diffuser. Diffusers that use a heat source (such as a light bulb ring) will alter the chemical make-up of the oil and its therapeutic qualities. A cold air diffuser uses room temperature air to blow the oil up against some kind of a nebulizer. This breaks the oil up into a micro-fine mist that is then dispersed into the air, covering hundreds of square feet in seconds. The oils, with their oxygenating molecules, will then remain suspended for several hours to freshen and improve the quality of the air. The antiviral, antibacterial, and antiseptic properties of the oils kill bacteria and help to reduce fungus and mold. Essential oils when diffused have been found to reduce the amount of airborne chemicals and metallics as well as help to create greater spiritual, physical, and emotional harmony. Diffusing oils for only 15 min. out of an hour gives the greatest therapeutic benefit as the olfactory system has time to recover before receiving more oils.
3. **Hot Water** - Put one to three drops of an essential oil into a bowl of hot water and inhale. Again, heat reduces some of the benefits.
4. **Vaporizer or Humidifier** - Put oil in a vaporizer or a humidifier. The cold air types are best since heat reduces some of the benefits.
5. **Fan or Vent** - Put oil on a cotton ball and attach to ceiling fans or air vents. This can also work well in a vehicle as the area is so small.

Baths

1. **Bath Water** - Begin by adding 3 to 6 drops of oil to the bath water while the tub is filling. Because the individual oils will separate as the water calms down, the skin will quickly draw the oils from the top of the water. People have commented that they were unable to endure more than 6 drops of oil. Such individuals may benefit from adding the oils to a bath and shower gel base first.

2. **Bath and Shower Gel** - Begin by adding three to 6 drops of oil to 1/2 oz. of a bath and shower gel base from Young Living or Dr. Woods castile soap and add to the water while the tub is filling. The number of drops can be increased as described above under bath water. Adding the oils to a bath and shower gel base first allows one to obtain the best benefit from the oils as they are more evenly dispersed throughout the water and not allowed to immediately separate.

3. **Wash Cloth** - When showering, add 3 to 6 drops of oil to a bath and shower gel base first before applying to a wash cloth to effectively cover the entire body.

STEAM DIFFUSION

Steam diffusion is a simple noninvasive home remedy to effectively deliver the life-giving qualities of Pure Grade unadulterated essential oils into the interstitial fluid, where it goes to work instantly, correcting cells and cleansing receptor sites, while bypassing the digestive tract and the skin. This is where the essential oil cleanses, oxygenates, and feeds the cells and tissues of the DNA blueprint.

An oil diffuser disperses the oil into the steam. The oil and the steam attract each other as one vapor. The heat in the steam will draw the blood to the surface. The baking soda will alkalize your system and when it comes in contact with the acid in your body, it produces carbon dioxide, which then causes the cells to increase respiration and pull in oxygen from the oil and moisture from the steam. The oxygen rich oils are delivered right into the cells from the interstitial fluid via the steam. This is an almost instant way of delivering the essential oils into the interstitial fluid via steam deep within the body where it starts to kill off bacteria and viruses and to feed the cells nutrients and oxygen.

Cells of the brain and the tissue of the body communicate by passing signals from one cell to another. Each cell has a place to receive the chemical that carries the message (called receptor sites). The chemical must cross the small space of interstitial fluid between each cell to be successful. In the interstitial fluid space, between the sending cell and the receiving cell, specific enzymes and nutrients affect the messages thereby having an effect on all the cells. These makeup your tissuse. Steam diffusion is very beneficial. It can be used at home for everything. It can be done as a family or by yourself.

The Recipe

To 1 qt. of distilled water, add one or a combination of the following:
- 1 tsp. sodium bicarbonate (aluminum free baking soda); helps with cancer and acidosis
- 1 tsp. potassium (cream of tartar); helps with depression
- 1 tsp. coral sea calcium powder helps with everything else

1. Bring calcium water to a slow even steam that vaporizes into the air. Add the desired oil into your diffuser and diffuse the oil straight into the steam. For therapeutic results throw a towel over your head and deeply inhale this steam for 15 min.
2. If you don't have a diffuser yet, drop 1 drop of oil directly into the boiling water every 3 min. When the oil hits the water, it vaporizes with the steam and the rest is scorched useless. That is why you need to drop 1 drop every 2 to 3 min.

Sodium Bicarbonate (Baking Soda) has been shown by Dr. Simoncini, M.D. to kill cancer-causing fungi within a matter of days. Go to livinganointed.com video section to see how to do the steam diffusion and for Dr. Simoncini info.

Go to www.livinganointed.com/videos.html to see how to do the steam diffusion and for Dr. Simoncini info

Why Choose Young Living Essential Oils?

Most of the oils on the market here in the United States are 4th and 5th quality oils, basically rejects from France. Many were originally produced for the perfume industry where they are distilled quickly at high pressure and high temperatures, fracturing the oil molecule and destroying the therapeutic qualities. Once brought to the United States, they are often cut with propylene glycol and synthetic constituents like lynelol acetate.

In order to have therapeutic effects, essential oils must be of the highest quality. They must be properly processed at low pressure and low temperature, they must be processed slowly and be free from added chemicals and solvents. Gary Young, founder of Young Living Essential Oils, built his own distiller and began distilling the plants grown for this purpose on his Idaho farm. Today, he is distilling some of the finest oils in the world! Young Living is committed to producing and selling the finest quality and purest oils in the world.

Knowing the Source

That is why it is so important to know the source of the essential oils you buy. Look for the European AFNOR or ISO certification - one of the most reliable indicators of essential oil quality. Find out if your supplier has each batch tested by several independent labs (in-house testing is very easily doctored). Check if the fragrances of the oils vary from batch to batch. If they've been distilled in small batches, rather than industrially processed (with chemicals and synthetic fragrance added), the fragrance should vary. Beware of cheap imitations and the health danger associated with adulterated oils! Here are excerpts from the 450-page book, *Essential Oils Desk Reference 4th Edition. You can purchase on LivingAnointed.com/eStore*

Where are these "Essential Oils" coming from?

In France, production of true lavender oil (Lavandula angustifolia) dropped from 87 tons in 1967 to only 12 tons in 1998. During this same period the demand for lavender oil grew over 100 percent. So where did essential oil marketers obtain enough lavender to meet demand? They probably used a combination of synthetic and adulterated oils. There are huge chemical companies on the east coast of the U.S. that specialize in the duplication of every essential oil that exists. For every kilogram of pure essential oil that is produced, it is estimated there are between 10 and 100 kilograms of synthetic oil created.

The one company in the world, who cares about the quality of its essential oils so much, that it would go through the effort of growing, harvesting, distilling, formulating, and marketing its oils, all under one roof: **Young Living Essential Oils!**

9 Essential Oils For Every Home and Everyday Use
With Young Living Essential Oils (YLEO)

- **Frankincense** - stimulating and elevating to the mind. Useful for visualizing, improving one's spiritual connection, and centering, it has comforting properties that help focus the mind and overcome stress and despair. Frankincense is considered holy anointing oil in the Middle East, where it has been used in religious ceremonies for thousands of years. I actually have some of the tree resin obtained from Gary Young.
- **Lavender** - the most versatile of all essential oils. Lavender is an adaptogen, and therefore can assist the body when adapting to stress or imbalances. This is a great aid for relaxing and winding down before bedtime. Balancing properties can also boost stamina and energy. It may be used to soothe and cleanse common cuts, bruises, and skin irritations.
- **Lemon** - powerful antioxidant. Strong, purifying, citrus scent is revitalizing, uplifting, and is a tonic for supporting the nervous and sympathetic system. A drop in a glass of water is delightfully refreshing and tastes great and may be beneficial for the skin.
- **PanAway** - soothing to the skin while providing comforting warmth to muscles after exercise. Often used for massage. Rub on temples, back of neck, or forehead, or inhale for a soothing effect. Use with a warm compress along the spine.
- **Peace and Calming** - helps calm tensions and uplift the spirit, promoting relaxation and a deep sense of peace. When massaged on the bottoms of the feet, it can be a wonderful prelude to a peaceful night's rest. It is calming and comforting to young children after an overactive and stressful day.
- **Peppermint** - most highly regarded herb for soothing digestion. It may also restore digestive efficiency. It has supportive effects on the liver and respiratory system. Improves concentration and mental sharpness. May directly affect the brain's satiety center, which triggers a sensation of fullness after meals.
- **Purification**- Can be used on the skin to cleanse/ sooth insect bites, scrapes and cuts. Diffusing will purify and cleanse the air from environmental impurities and odors. Put on cotton ball and place in air vents of home, car, hotel room and office.
- **Thieves** - was created based on research about four thieves in France who covered themselves with Cloves, Rosemary, Cinnamon Bark, Lemon, and Eucalyptus while robbing plague victims. Tested for its cleansing abilities. This is highly effective in supporting the immune system and good health.
- **Valor** - empowering combination of therapeutic grade essential oils working with both the physical and spiritual aspects of the body to increase feelings of strength, courage, and selfesteem in the face of adversity. Strengthening. Enhances internal resources. Also found to help alignment in the body.

Top Unwanted Toxic Chemicals Found In Your Home

This list is to be used for all substances in your home i.e food, drink, skin/hair care, cleaners etc. These chemical have been verified by the EPA or Material Safety Data Sheet (MSDS) as hazardous or cancerous. This list is growing daily. Check the livinganointed.com for an updated cheat sheet. You can go to google, type in the chemical name, then MSDS science lab. There you can read the report and make your own decisions. Be your own health advocate.

Chemical Name	Description & Side Effects
1,4-dioxano	Used as stabilizer in solvents such as personal care products, cleaners, dyes, make up, oils, dry cleaning chemical, varnishes, paints, plastics. Causes cancer in animals. It is considered a probable human carcinogen by the U.S. Environmental Protection Agency and the WHOIA. Affect you through <u>inhalation, skin absorption, and ingestion</u>. It is an <u>eye, respiratory tract irritant, mucous membrane & skin irritant, central nervous system depressant</u>. Causes damage to the liver and kidneys.
2-bromo-2-nitropropane-1,3-diol (Bronopol)	"Toxic, causes allergic contact dermatitis. See Nitrosating agents
Acesuifame K, Ace K,	See Aspartame
Alcohol (Isopropyl) & SD-40	As a **solvent and denaturant** (a poisonous substance that changes another substance's natural qualities), alcohol is made from propylene, a petroleum derivative. A petroleum-derived substance, it is also used in antifreeze and as a solvent in shellac and diluted essential oils. According to A Consumer's Dictionary of Cosmetic Ingredients, ingestion or inhalation of the vapor may cause headaches, flushing dizziness, mental depressions, nausea, vomiting, narcosis, anaesthesia, and coma. The fatal ingested dose is one ounce. A very drying and irritating solvent and dehydrator that strips your skin's natural acid mantle, making us more vulnerable to bacteria, molds and viruses. It may promote brown spots and premature aging of skin. Used in personal care products, mouthwash, toners, baby products.
AMMONIUM's Bicarbonate or Hydrogen, Acid Ammonium Carbonate, Monoammonium Salt & Carbonate	Ammonium bicarbonate (A.B.) is used in dyes, pigments, it is also a basic for fertilizer, widely used in the plastic and rubber industry, in ceramics, fire-extinguishing, pharmaceutical & tanning. A.B. is an irritant to the skin, eyes and respiratory system.
Ammonium laureth or Lauryl Sulfate (ALS)	**See Anionic Surfactants**
Aniline	Related to both benzene and ammonia, it is used to make a wide variety of organic chemical compounds including pharmaceuticals, photographic chemicals, and dye intermediates. **See Benzene**

Chemical Name	Description & Side Effects
Anionic Surfactants	They are a negatively charged ion and they may be contaminated with nitrosamines, which are carcinogenic. Used as **detergents and surfactants**, yet are used as one of the major ingredients in about 90% of all **products that foam**. The American College of Toxicology (ACT) states they can cause malformation in children's eyes and may be damaging to the immune system, especially within the skin. Skin layers may separate and inflame due to its protein denaturing properties. It is possibly the most dangerous of all ingredients in personal care products. Research has shown that **SLS** when combined with other chemicals can be transformed into nitrosamines, a potent class of carcinogens, which cause the body to absorb nitrates at higher levels than eating nitrate-contaminated food. (ACT) report, SLS stays in the body for up to five days and easily penetrates through the skin and enters and maintains residual levels in the heart, liver, lungs, brain, and swelling of the skin in a allergic reaction. Used in car washes, garage floor cleaners, engine degreaser, dishwashing detergents, and 90% of personal care products.
Antibacteriales	Antibacterial agents such as Triclosan (hand purifier, 2 oz is = to 4 shots of vodka) encourage the rise of drug-resistant bacteria. Used in cleansers, deodorants, cosmetics. **See Triclosan**
Artificial Coloring	Synthetic top of the list goes to Tartrazine 102. It causes flare-ups of allergies, sensitivity reactions and so many bad side effects that no one should consider swallowing it, let alone feed it to a child! Artificial colors, such as Blue 1 and Green 3, are carcinogenic. D&C Red 33, FD&C Yellow 5, and FD&C yellow 6 have been shown to cause cancer not only when ingested, but also when applied to the skin. The use of permanent or semi permanent hair color products, particularly black and dark brown colors, is associated with increased incidence of human cancer. Contributes to hyperactivity in children; may contribute to learning and visual disorders, nerve damage. When people senistive to #5 eat food that contains Yellow #5, they suffer from hives, a runny or stuffy nose, & occasionally, breathing difficulties. Used in food, drinks, make-up, toothpaste, mouthwash shampoos, hair dyes.

Chemical Name	Description & Side Effects
Aspartame NutraSweet, Equal, sucralose (Splenda), neotame, saccharin, Sweet 'N Low, Sweet One, acesulfame-k, Sunette, Sweet-n-Safe	One out of 20,000 babies is born with phenylketonuria (PKU), which means it is unable to safely tolerate phenylalanine--one of the two amino acids contained in aspartame. If too much phenylalanine accumulates in the blood of a baby with PKU (can happen even before birth), it can result in mental retardation. Because of the PKU problem, the FDA requires all packaged foods that contain aspartame to carry a warning. Some scientists are concerned might cause altered brain function & behavioral changes. Hundreds of people have said they suffer from dizziness, headaches, epileptic-like seizures, and menstrual problems after using the sweetener. Dr. Louis Elsas, told Congress that aspartame could cause neurological damage in children & passing from pregnant mothers to their unborn child, affecting brain development. It breaks down in the body to phenylalanine (a neurotoxin that cause seizures), aspartic acid (damages the developing brain) & methanol (turns into formaldehyde). Crosses the placental barrier from mother to baby. Implicated in diseases such as multiple sclerosis & Non-Hodgkin's Lymphoma. **See Aspartame Doc.**
Benzalkonium chloride	**See Cationic Surfactants**. Highly toxic, primary skin irritant
Benzene	Benzene and the other aromatic hydrocarbons are obtained for industrial purposes from the distillation of coal tar, a byproduct in the manufacture of coke, and from petroleum by special reforming methods. Natural sources of benzene include volcanoes, forest fires, crude oil, gasoline, and cigarette smoke. It is highly flammable. Benzene is a known carcinogen and cause cancer and central nervous system toxicity, leukemia, anemia, a malignant disease that affects the blood and bone marrow by causing anemia and depressed immune function. In chronic poisoning the onset is slow, with the symptoms: fatigue, headache, dizziness, nausea and loss of appetite, loss of weight, and weakness. Benzene is easily absorbed into the bloodstream through the inhalation of vapors and mist. It can also be absorbed through your skin and into your bloodstream when in contact with a person's body. Used in plastics, resins, nylon, synthetic fibers, some types of rubbers, lubricants, dyes, detergents, drugs, pesticides.
Benzoic acid, 210, 211, 219	This product causes hyperactive reactions in susceptible people, skin rashes, and makes asthma bouts worse. It is one of the worst additives for setting off reactions. They can cause severe contact dermatitis or redness, swelling, itching, skin pain, asthma attacks and anaphylactic shock in susceptible persons.

Chemical Name	Description & Side Effects
Butylated Hydroxyanisole **(BHA)** 320, Butylated Hydroxytoluene **(BHT)** 321	These two closely related chemicals are added to **prevent oxidation and retard rancidity in oil-containing foods**. The State of California has listed it as a carcinogen. Some studies show the same cancer causing possibilities for BHT 321. The bottom line is that BHA and BHT are unnecessary. Propyl gallate, is closely related to BHA and BHT. Banned in England, is associated with <u>liver and kidney damage, behavioral problems, infertility, weakened immune system, birth defects and cancer</u>. **See benzene.**
Bis-2-ethylhexyl sodiumsulfosuccinate	See Dioctyl sodium sulfosuccinate
Bisphenol-A (BPA)	Adverse health effects from BPA include; early puberty, breast cancer, diabetes, low sperm count, obesity, attention deficit disorder, brain damage, endocrine disruption, miscarriage, and cancer." BPA is a chemical that is used to make polycarbonate plastic, a lightweight, heat-resistant & durable plastic. It is found in most plastic bottles, containers, line metal food cans, white dental sealants, baby bottles & in some children toys. The Centers for Disease Control states that 95% of Americans have detectable levels of BPA in their bodies. BPA interacts with estrogen receptors within the cell nucleus and mimics estrogen by attaching to the cells' estrogen receptors. BPA exposure in utero can lead to abnormal brain & reproductive development.

Chemical Name	Description & Side Effects
Brominated Vegetable Oil (BVO)	Linked to <u>major organ system damage, birth defects, growth problems</u>; considered <u>unsafe by the FDA</u>, can still lawfully be used unless further action is taken by the FDA . Used to give long shelf life. BVO is vegetable oil that has had atoms of the element bromine bonded to it and is used as an **emulsifier** in citrus-flavored drinks to help <u>natural fat-soluble citrus flavors stay suspended in the drink and to produce a cloudy appearance</u>. The BVO remains suspended in the drink instead of forming separate layers. In Mountain Dew, Gatorade, Powerade, Mello Yello, Pineapple, Orange Fanta, Sun Drop, Squirt, Fresca. In test animals, traces remain in the body fat and causes damage to the heart and kidneys in addition to increasing fat deposits in these organs. Bromine is a BVO displaces iodine, which may depress thyroid function. Evidence for this has been extrapolated from pre-1975 cases where bromine-containing sedatives resulted in emergency room visits and incorrect diagnoses of psychosis and brain damage due to side effects; depression, memory loss, hallucinations, violent tendencies, seizures, cerebral atrophy, acute irritability, tremors, ataxia, confusion, loss of peripheral vision, slurred speech, stupor, tendon reflex changes, photophobia due to enlarged pupils, & extensor plantar responses. In extreme cases BVO has caused testicular damage, stunted growth and produced lethargy and fatigue.
Bronopol 2-bromo 2-nitropropano -1, 3 diol	May break down in products into formaldehyde and also cause the formation of carcinogenic nitrosamines under certain conditions. Most expensive lines of cosmetics and baby products us this chemical.
Butylene Glycol	**See Propylene Glycol**
Caffeine	Caffeine is found naturally in tea, coffee, and cocoa. It is one of the few drugs - a stimulant - added to foods, drinks, candy etc. <u>Caffeine increases stomach acid</u> and may cause peptic ulcers, raise blood pressure temporarily, and makes some blood vessels open wider and others to narrow. "Caffeine intake causes symptoms ranging from nervousness to insomnia in any age. Caffeine may also interfere with reproduction and affect developing fetuses. Experiments on lab animals link caffeine to birth defects such as cleft palates, missing fingers and toes, and skull malformations." Caffeine is addictive, and some people experience headaches when they stop drinking it. *mindfully.org http://www.healthofchildren.com/C/Caffeine.html*
Carbomer	**See Benzene**

Chemical Name	Description & Side Effects
Cationic Surfactants /Ammoniums	These chemicals have a positive electrical charge. They contain a quaternary ammonium group and are often called "quats". These are used in hair conditioners, but originated from the paper and fabric industries as softeners and anti-static agents. In the long run they cause the hair to become dry and brittle. They are synthetic, irritating, allergenic and toxic, and oral intake of them can be lethal.
Ceteareths	Contaminated with the volatile carcinogens ethylene oxide and dioxane
Cetrimonium Cloride	**See Cationic Surfactants**
Cetylpyridinium chloride or bromide, cepacol, ceprim, cepacol chloride, cetafilm, cetamium, dobendan, medilave, asept, ercocet	It is an antiseptic that kills bacteria and other microorganisms. This is in certain pesticides. Cause brown stains between the teeth. Concentrated solutions are destructive to mucous membranes. It is very toxic when inhaled. It is also combustible. Used in mouthwashes, toothpastes, lozenges, throat sprays, anti-snore, breath & nasal sprays.
Chloromethylisothiazolin	Causes contact dermatitis
Chlorine	Exposure to chlorine in tap water, showers, pools, laundry products, cleaning agents, food processing, sewage systems and many other sources, can affect health by contributing to asthma, hay fever, anemia, bronchitis, circulatory collapse, confusion, delirium, diabetes, dizziness, irritation of the eye, mouth, nose, throat, lung, skin and stomach, heart disease, high blood pressure and nausea. It is also a possible cause of cancer.
Coal Tars	Coal tar is a brown or black liquid of high viscosity, which smells of naphthalene and aromatic hydrocarbons. Coal tar is among the by-products when coal is carbonized to make coke or gasified to make coal gas. Coal tars are complex and variable mixtures of phenols, polycyclic aromatic hydrocarbons (PAHs), and heterocyclic compounds. Used in Hair /skin care, hair dyes, soap, food, drinks, cosmetics. **See Phenols.**
Cocoamidopropyl Betaine	Can cause eye and skin irriation
Cocoyl Sarcosine	**See Anionic Surfactants**
DEA (diethanolamine), Oleamide, Stearamide, DEA-Cetyl Phosphate, Oleth-3 Phosphate, Lauramide, Linoleamide, **MEA** (Monoethanolamine) Myristamide, ocamide DEA or MEA **TEA** (triethanolamine), TEA-Lauryl Sulfate	**Function as emulsifiers or foaming agents.** These chemicals are hormone-disrupting chemicals known to form nitrates and nitrosamines. A Federal government study says that DEA and DEA-based detergents have been shown to greatly increase the risk of cancer, especially liver and kidney cancer. DEA-related ingredients are widely used in a variety of cosmetic products. Used in shampoos, body washes, shaving cream, moisturizers, cosmetics, deodorant, toothpaste. *http://vm.cfsan.fda.gov/~dms/cos-dea.html*

Chemical Name	Description & Side Effects
Diazolidinyl Urea	Established as a primary cause of contact dermatitis (American Academy of Dermatology). Contains formaldehyde, a <u>carcinogenic chemical, is toxic by inhalation, a strong irritant, and causes contact dermatitis</u>. Causes severe eye & skin irritation. Contact causes burning sensaton, inflammation, burns, profound damage to tissue. Reports have suggested that Diazolidinyl Urea (D.U) is a formaldehyde releaser. Used in cosmetic and personal care products.
Dioctyl Sodium Sulfosuccinate	Toxicity to humans, including carcinogenicity, reproductive and developmental toxicity, neurotoxicity, and acute toxicity. Toxicity to aquatic organisms. Severe eye irritation. Skin irritation. Ingestion causes diarrhea, intestinal bloating, cramps, nausea. Used in constipation medications, used on dogs and cats to control fleas, insecticides, rodenticides, and cool aid packets and drinks.
Dioxins	Dioxins contain surfactants or detergents. They are highly volatile 1,4 – dioxane, which is both <u>readily inhaled and absorbed through the skin</u>. The Consumer Product Safety Commission concluded that "the presence of 1,4 – dioxane, even as a trace contaminant, is a cause of concern." These avoidable risks of cancer in numerous personal care, and other consumer products, is inexcusable, particularly as the dioxane is readily removed from surfactants during their manufacture by a process known as "vacuum stripping." Used in personal care products and household products.
Disodium Sulfosuccinate	**See Anionic Surfactants**
DMDM Hydantoin	**See formaldehyde.**
EDTA	**See Tetrasodium Pyrophosphate**
Formaldehyde, DMDM Hydantoin, Diazolidinyl Urea, Quaternium-16	<u>Formaldehyde is a known carcinogen (causes cancer)</u>. Causes allergic, irritant and contact dermatitis, headaches and chronic fatigue. The vapour is extremely irritating to the eyes, nose and throat (mucous membranes). According to the Mayo Clinic, formaldehyde can irritate the respiratory system, cause skin reactions and trigger heart palpitations. <u>Exposure to formaldehyde may cause joint pain, allergies, depression, headaches, chest pains, ear infections, chronic fatigue, dizziness and loss of sleep.</u> It can also aggravate coughs and colds and trigger asthma. Serious side effects include <u>weakening of the immune system and cancer</u>. It can be absorbed through the skin and nails. Used in Found in eye shadows, mascaras cosmetics, antiperspirants, nail polish, perfumes, oral jel, almost all skin care products.

Chemical Name	Description & Side Effects
Fragrance	Fragrance on a label can indicate the presence of up to four thousand separate ingredients, many toxic or carcinogenic. Symptoms reported to the US FDA include headaches, dizziness, allergic rashes, skin discoloration, violent coughing and vomiting, and skin irritation. Clinical observation proves fragrances can affect the central nervous system, causing depression, hyperactivity, irritability and inability to cope, and other behavioral changes. Used in many personal care and baby products, candles, plug-ins, and essential oils.
Guarana	Each Guarana fruit contains a seed, which contains approx. 3 times as much caffeine as coffee beans.
Glycol Ethers- EGPE, EGME, EGEE, DEGBE, PGME, DPGME	Widely used industrial solvents found in nail polish, deodorant, perfumes and other cosmetics, some glycol ethers are hazardous to the reproductive system. Other effects of overexposure include anemia and irritation of the skin, eyes, nose and throat.
HIGH-FRUCTOSE CORN SYRUP "corn sweetener," "corn syrup," or "corn syrup solids"	High-fructose corn syrup is beginning to suggest that this liquid sweetener may upset the human metabolism, raising the risk for heart disease and diabetes. Researchers say that high-fructose corn syrup's chemical structure encourages overeating. It also seems to force the liver to pump more heart-threatening triglycerides into the bloodstream. In addition, fructose may zap your body's reserves of chromium, a mineral important for healthy levels of cholesterol, insulin, and blood sugar.
Imidazolidinyl urea	Releases formaldehyde, a carcinogenic chemical, into cosmetics at over temperatures 10°C. Toxic. **See Formaldehyde**
Isobutane	Very toxic by inhalation. Very toxic in contact with skin. Very toxic if swallowed. When commonly sold as fuel, it is also known as liquified petroleum gas (LPG or LP-gas) and can be a mixture of propane with smaller amounts of propylene, butane, and butylene.
Isothiazolinone	Contact dermatitis, corrosive to the eyes, skin and mucous membranes and the lungs. Can cause allergic reactions.
Lead	Lead damages the nervous system, leading to decreased learning ability and behavioral deficits. Reproductive toxin. Carcinogen. [Strong animal, human and children evidence] (used as a preservative) Used in Hair dyes- Grecian formula, eye makeup.
Lanolin	Any chemicals used on sheep will contaminate the lanolin obtained from the wool. The majority of lanolin used in cosmetics is highly contaminated with pesticides and insecticides. Lanolin itself is perfectly safe. But cosmetic-grade lanolin can be contaminated with carcinogenic pesticides such as DDT, and other neurotoxic pesticides.
Lauryl dimonium hydrolysed collagen	**See Cationic Surfactants**
Liquidum Paraffinum	**See Mineral Oil**
Mercury	A brain and nervous system toxin as well as a known carcinogen and hormone disruptor. It is found in lead acetate in hair dyes, makeup, and vaccines.

Chemical Name

Description & Side Effects

Chemical Name	Description & Side Effects
Methylpropane	**See Isobutane**
Methanol / Formaldehyde	**See Aspartame.** Approximately 10% of aspartame (by mass) is broken down into methanol in the small intestine. Most of the methanol is absorbed and quickly converted into formaldehyde. Alleged harmful effects of aspartame ingestion include seizures and a change in the level of dopamine, a brain neurotransmitter. Symptoms associated with lupus, multiple sclerosis, and Alzheimer's disease have been claimed to result from an excess intake of aspartame.
Mineral Oil	Baby oil is 100% mineral oil which is petroleum. This ingredient actually coats the skin just like plastic wrap, clogging the pores and disrupting the skin's natural immune barrier and inhibiting its ability to breathe and absorb the Natural Moisture Factor. As the body's largest organ of elimination, it is vital that the skin be free to release toxins. Mineral oil impedes the elimination process, allowing toxins to accumulate, which can promote acne, clogging of pores and other disorders. Any mineral oil derivative can be contaminated with cancer causing PAH's (Polycyclic Aromatic Hydrocarbons). Used in many personal care products and some foods.
Miralax	See Polyethylene Glycol (PEG) - used before you have an colonoscopy. Golytely7, Colyte7, Nulytely7, OCL7, Trilyte, Halflytely, PEG 3350
Modified Starches	Modified starches are used in processed foods to improve their consistency and keep the solids suspended. Often starch and modified starch replace large amounts of nutritious ingredients, such as fruits. Starch thickened baby foods contain 75% less fruit than 100% fruit baby foods. Modified starches 1400 to 1450 can cause diarrhea in babies. Babies cannot digest starch and should not be treated to a chemical cocktail in baby food.
Monosodium Glutamate, MSG, 622	MSG - may cause headaches, itching, nausea, nervous system, depression, anger, agatation, reproductive disorders, and high blood pressure. Other names for MSG, Autolyzed Plant Protein, Autolyzed Yeast, Calcium Caseinate, Gelatin, Glutamate, Glutamic Acid, Hydrolyzed Oat Flour, Hydrolyzed Plant Protein (HPP), Hydrolyzed Protein, Hydrolyzed Vegetable Protein (HVP), Monopotassium Glutamate, Monosodium Glutamate, Natrium Glutamate, Plant Protein Extract, Sodium Caseinate, Textured Protein, Yeast Extract, Yeast Food or Nutrient. Used in infant formula, low fat milk, candy, chewing gum, drinks, foods, skin care, medications.
Neotame	Similar to aspartame, but potentially more toxic; awaiting approval. A dangerous excitotoxin.

Chemical Name	Description & Side Effects
Nitrite and Nitrate	Sodium nitrite and sodium nitrate have been used for centuries to preserve meat. They maintain the red color, contribute to the flavor, and inhibit the growth of botulism-causing bacteria. Nitrate is harmless, but it is easily converted -by bacteria in foods and in the body- to nitrite. When nitrite combines with compounds called secondary amines, it forms powerful cancer-causing nitrosamines. Nitrosamine formation occurs most readily at the high temperatures of frying, but may also take place in the stomach. Use nitrite-free processed meats~**See Nitrite Doc.**
Olestra	Causes gastrointestinal irritation, reduces carotenoids and fat soluble vitamins in the body. The side effects from it can be fatal because it drags valuable nutrients out of the body as it passes through. Some of the nutrients it steals are ones that protect the body from such diseases as lung cancer, prostate cancer, heart disease, and macular degeneration.
Paraben (methyl, propyl, butyl, ethyl)	Used to extend shelf life of products. Widely used even though they are known to be toxic. Have caused many allergic reactions and skin rashes. Highly toxic. The estrogenic activity of parabens may be linked to the development of breast cancer. These preservatives have the ability to mimic estrogen in the body. Parabens may be absorbed through pregnant women's skin, where they then may act as an alien female hormone. A male exposed to this hormone as a fetus may develop fertility problems as an adult. Used in 99 percent of all cosmetic and body care products, and vitamins.
Paraffin wax or oil	**See Mineral Oil**
Partially Hydrogenated vegetable oils	Associated with heart disease, breast and colon cancer, atherosclerosis, elevated cholesterol, depressed immune system, allergies.
PEG	**See polyethylene glycol.** That is used in making cleansers to dissolve oil and grease. Strips the Natural Moisture Factor, leaving the immune system vulnerable and are potentially carcinogenic.
Petrolatum (Vaseline)	**See Mineral Oil.**
Phenol	**See Benzene.** Its chief uses are in the manufacturing of plastics, dyes, and disinfectants.
Phenylenediamine (PPD)	Linked with skin irritations, and respiratory disorders. PPD is mutagenic and reasonably anticipated to be a human carcinogen, and has been banned in Europe. Also called oxidation dyes, amino dyes, para dyes, or peroxide dyes. Used in hairdyes.

Chemical Name	Description & Side Effects
Phenylketonuria (PKU)	PKU is an autosomal recessive genetic disorder characterized by a deficiency in the enzyme phenylalanine hydroxylase (PAH). This enzyme is necessary to metabolize the amino acid phenylalanine into the amino acid tyrosine. When PAH is deficient, phenylalanine accumulates and is converted into phenylketones, which are detected in the urine. Left untreated, this condition can cause problems with brain development, leading to progressive hyperactivity, EEG abnormalities and seizures, and severe mental retardation, albinism (excessively fair hair and skin), a tendency to hypopigmentation and eczema are major clinical problems later in life. Is an by-product of aspartame brake down.
Phthalates DBP, DMP, DEP	Toxic gender bending chemical used as a plasticizer in food wraps, pliable plastics. It is readily absorbed into the bodys system. Phthalates are implicated as causing low sperm counts, and sexual abnormalities and deformities. _www.health-report. co.uk._ They are used because the oily texture of phthalates acts like a moisturizer & helps lotions penetrate skin. Endocrine disruption; cell line transformations; and cancers, including those of the liver, kidney, and mononuclear cell leukemia. Used in fragrances, deodorants, nail polishes, hair products, lotions, plastics, and cosmetics.
Plastics	**See Toxic Plastics** Bottles and Containers documents. AVOID using #3, #6, and #7
Poloxamer 407	**See poly-propylene glycol** - contact lens solutions, mouthwash, cosmetics
Polyethylene Gycol (PEG) and poly-ethylene oxide (PEO)	This is used in **cleansers to dissolve oil and grease as well as to thicken products.** A number after "PEG" refers to its molecular weight, which influences its characteristics. Because of their effectiveness, PEGs are often used in caustic spray-on oven cleaners, yet are also found in many personal care products. Not only are they potentially carcinogenic, but they contribute to stripping the skin's Natural Moisture Factor, leaving the immune system vulnerable. Used in make-up, hair products, lotions, after-shave, deodorants, mouthwashes and toothpaste. **See Propylene Glycol.**
Potassium Bromate	Can cause nervous system, kidney disorders, and gastrointestinal upset; may be carcinogenic.
Potassium Coco Hydrolyzed Collagen	**See Anionic Surfactants**
Propane	**See Isobutane**

Chemical Name	Description & Side Effects
Propylene Glycol (PG) Butylene Glycol PROPANEDIOL, DIHYDROXY-PROPANE, METHYLETHYLENE GLYCOL, PROPANE	(PG) is a petroleum derivative. PG is actually the active component in antifreeze. There is no difference between what is used in industry and what is used in personal care products. Industry uses it to **break down protein and cellular structure (what the skin is made of**. Because of PG's ability to quickly penetrate the skin, the EPA requires workers to wear protective gloves, clothing, and goggles when working with this toxic substance. PG's MSDS warn against skin contact because PG has systemic consequences, such as brain, liver, and kidney abnormalities. It penetrates the skin and can weaken protein and cellular structure. PG is strong enough to remove barnacles from boats! Health Hazard Acute and Chronic. May cause respiratory and throat irritation, central nervous system depression, blood and kidney disorders, Nystagmus, Lymphocytosis, skin & eye irritation, dermatitis, and the list goes on. Used in Skin care, hair products, oral products, food & drinks.

NOTE: visit LivingAnointed.com to print out Anti-Freeze container showing the name Propylene Glycol. I actually have the container proving this. It is really hard to find the Low Tox Anti-Freeze containers anymore. |
PVP/VA Copolymer	**See Mineral Oil.** Toxic since particles may contribute to foreign bodies in the lungs. A petroleum-derived chemical. It can be considered toxic, since particles may contribute to foreign bodies in the lungs of sensitive persons. Used in hairsprays, wavesets, and cosmetics.
Quaternium-7, 15, 31, 60, etc	See formaldehyde. Toxic, causes skin rashes and allergic reactions. Formaldehyde releasers. Substantive evidence of casual relationship to leukemia, multiple myeloma, non-Hodgkin's lymphoma and other cancers.
Saccharin, 954	Use of this product may be hazardous to your health. Several studies linked it to cancer in laboratory animals. 350 times sweeter than sugar. Might interfere with blood coagulation, blood sugar levels and digestive function. Causes cancer of the bladder, uterus, ovaries, skin and blood vessels in animals. Has been linked to DNA damage and congenital abnormalities in animals. May contribute to obesity. A dangerous excitotoxin. Used in Medications, vitamins, foods, and drinks.
Silica	Specifically amorphous hydrated silica, may be contaminated with small amounts of crystalline quartz. Crystalline silica is carcinogenic.
Silicone derived emollients	Silicone emollients are occlusive - that is they coat the skin, trapping anything beneath it, and do not allow the skin to breathe (much like plastic wrap would do.)

Chemical Name	Description & Side Effects
Sodium Benzoate	The substance may be toxic to blood, the reproductive system, liver, and the central nervous system (CNS). Repeated or prolonged exposure to the substance can produce organ damage. Commonly used in soft drinks, meat products, baked goods.
Sodium Cocoyl Sarcosinate, Sodium	Sodium Laureth Sulfate (SLES), Sodium Lauryl Sulfate (SLS), Sodium Lauryl Sarcosinate, Sodium Methyl Cocoyl Taurate. **See Anionic Surfactants**
Sodium dioctyl sulfosuccinate	**See Dioctyl sodium sulfosuccinate**
Sodium Hexametaphosphate	Toxicity to humans, including carcinogenicity, reproductive and developmental toxicity, neurotoxicity. Hazardous in case of ingestion. May cause skin irritation, eye irritation, respiratory tract irritation, coughing, shortness of breath, gastrointestinal tract irritation with nausea, vomiting, and diarrhea. May affect behavior/central nervous system/peripheral nervous system, urinary system, and (kidneys- renal failure). It may also cause heart disturbances (fall in blood pressure, slow pulse). The toxicity of phosphates results from their ability to sequester calcium. Systemic metabolic acidosis may result as this material is believed to be hydrolyzed into ortho phosphates when ingested (before absorption). Tetany (mineral imbalance in the body, results in severe muscle spasms). Used in drinks, Sunny Delight, Hawaiian punch, tooth paste, foods, chemicals and pesticides.
Sodium Hydroxide	Also known as caustic soda. Workers exposed to steam containing sodium hydroxide have suffered lung damage and an increased risk of throat cancer. Causes contact dermatitis and sensitizes individuals to other chemicals. POISONOUS! CORROSIVE. May be fatal if swallowed, harmful if inhaled, causes burns to any area of contact. Used in drains, pipes, oven cleaners, toothpastes, food, skin care.
Sodium Hydroxymethylglycinate	Causes moderate skin, and eye irritation. May cause an allergic skin reaction.
ANY - Sodium **Laureth** or **Lauryl** SLES or SLS Sulfate	**See Anionic Surfactants**
Sodium Methyl Cocoyl	**See Anionic Surfactants**
Stearalkonium Chloride	**See Cationic Surfactants**
Succinic acid	This acid is combustible and corrosive, capable of causing burns. "Harmful by inhalation, ingestion and through skin absorption. Wash after handling. Eye contact may cause serious damage." Used in pharmaceuticals, vitamins, and perfumes.
Sucralose (Splenda)	**See Aspartame Doc.** Tests reveal it can cause up to 40% shrinkage of the thymus gland, and causes swelling of the kidneys and liver, liver calcification, and weight gain. Splenda has basically been chlorinated. The sugar molecule has now been transformed into a chlorocarbon - a chemical agent that has no place in the human diet.

Chemical Name	Description & Side Effects
Sulfites	"Sulfites" are a class of chemicals that can keep cut fruits and vegetables looking fresh. They also prevent discoloration in apricots, raisins, and other dried fruits; control "black spot" in freshly caught shrimp; and prevent discoloration, bacterial growth, and fermentation in wine. Sulfites could provoke sever allergic reactions. The FDA identified at least a dozen fatalities linked to sulfites. All of the deaths occurred among asthmatics. If you have asthma, be sure to consider whether your attacks might be related to sulfites. Destroys vitamin B1; small amounts may cause asthma, anaphylactic shock; dangerous for asthma, allergy sufferers; has caused deaths.
Sulphur dioxide	This preservative is commonly used in beer, wine, soft drinks and dried fruits to stop them from fermenting. Asthmatics may suffer an attack after inhaling sulphur dioxide and it has also been linked to stomach upsets. An ongoing review by the WHO Expert Committee on Food Additives confirmed sulphur dioxide could destroy vitamin B1, so having a soft drink with your meal could wipe out its vitamin B1 content. The same review found that animal and lab tests revealed that consuming E220 could increase the amount of calcium lost by the body - raising your risk of the bone-thinning condition osteoporosis - and could cause DNA damage. Used in soft drinks, dried fruit, juices, potato products, foods.
Sweet 'N Low	Contains saccharin. **See Aspartame.** A dangerous excitotoxin.
Talc	Scientific studies have shown that routine application of talcum powder in the genital area is associated with a three-to-fourfold increase in the development of ovarian cancer. Acute or chronic lung disease (Talcosis). Used in make up, baby and foot powder, anti acids, and medications.
TEA (Triethanolamine)	**See Anionic Surfactants & Laureth Sulfate. Highly acidic**
Tartrazine 102	**See Artificial Coloring**
Tetra - anything	**See Tetrasodium Pyrophoshate EDTA**
Tetrasodium Pyrophoshate EDTA Tetrasodium anything	Exposure to tetrasodium pyrophosphate causes irritation in humans. It is an alkaline chemical and acute exposures have resulted in mild to moderate irritation of the eyes, skin, nose, throat, and respiratory passages. EDTA is synthetic and not found naturally. There is concern that EDTA may deplete important vitamins and minerals.

Chemical Name	Description & Side Effects
Titanium dioxide	It is metal that is corrosion-resistant (to sea water and chlorine). It has the functions of sterilization, antibacterium, deodorization, moldproof, algaproof, antirust, fadeproof, self-cleaning and antifouling. Titanium dioxide powder brings photochemical reaction through ultraviolet radiation and daylight, etc. It can directly decompose contacted organic materials (formaldehyde, ammonia, benzene), bacterium, viruses, odors and anaphylactic materials in the air and in the water. Used in paints, plastics, papers, inks, foods, coloring, toothpastes, cosmetic, tattos, drinking water and sewage treatment.
Toluene	**See benzene.** A solvent, able to dissolve paint & thinners, rubber, ink, glues, lacquers, leather tanners, disinfectants. POSON! Harmful if inhaled, absorbed through skin or swallowed. Endocrine disruptor, potential carcinogen may cause birth defects, irritates respiratory tract, may cause liver damage.
Triclosan	The EPA registers it as a pesticide, risk to both human health and the environment. It is a chlorinated aromatic, similar in molecular structure and chemical formula to some of the most toxic chemicals on earth: dioxins, PCB's, and Agent Orange. Hormone disruptors pose enormous long-term chronic health risks because they interfere with the way hormones perform (changing genetic material, or fostering birth defects). Triclosan is a chlorophenol, a class of chemicals suspected of causing cancer in humans. Externally, it can cause skin irritations, stored in body fat, accumulate to toxic levels, and damaging the liver, kidneys, and lungs, and can cause paralysis, sterility, suppression of immune function, brain hemorrhaging, decreased fertility and sexual function, heart problems, and coma. A antibiotic agent such as triclosan used everyday will destroy the beneficial bacteria in our bodies. Used in antibacterial chemicals, detergents, dish soaps, laundry soaps, deodorants, cosmetics, personal care.
Urea (Imidazolidinyl)	**See Formaldehyde doc**

For more information please visit LivingAnointed.com

Toxic Chemical Cheat Sheet

This list is to be used for all products in your home I.e food, drink, body care, cleaners etc. These chemicals have been verified by the EPA, OSHA or Material Safety Data Sheet (MSDS) as hazardous. This list is growing daily, check the LivingAnointed.com for updates. You can go to Google, type in the chemical name then MSDS. Then you can read the report and make your own decisions. Be your own health advocate, don't assume... Research!

1,4-dioxane	Flavor (s), Flavoring(s)	Polyethylene oxide (PEO)
2,4-dione	Formaldehyde	Potassium Bromate
5,5-dimethylimidazolidine	Fragrance	Potassium Coco Hydrolyzed Collagen
Acesuifame K, Ace K,	Glutamate	Propane (any)
Acid Ammonium Carbonate	Glutamic Acid	Propylene Glycol (PG)
Alcohol (Isopropyl) & SD-40	Glycol Ethers	Protease enzymes
Ammonium Laureth/ Lauryl Sulfate (ALS)	Go Lite drink	PVP/VA Copolymer
AMMONIUM's Bicarbonate or Hydrogen	Guarana	Quaternium-7, 15, 31, 60, etc
Aniline	Hexametaphosphate	Saccharin, 954
Anionic Surfactants	High Fructose Corn Syrup	Silica
Antibacterials	Hydrolyzed (anything)	Silicone derived emollients
Anything protein fortified	Imidazolidinyl urea	Sodium Caseinate
Artificial Coloring	Iodopropynyl	Sodium Cocoyl Sarcosinate
Asept	Isobutane	Sodium dioctyl sulfosuccinate
Aspartame	Isothiazolinone	Sodium Hexametaphosphate
Autolyzed (anything)	Lanolin	Sodium Hydroxide
Azodicarbonamide	Lauryl dimonium hydrolysed collagen	Sodium Hydroxymethylglycinate
Barley malt	Lead	Sodium Laureth Sulfate (SLES)
Benzalkonium chloride	Liquidum Paraffinum	Sodium Lauryl Sarcosinate
Benzene	Malt extract or flavoring	Sodium Lauryl Sulfate (SLS)
Benzoic acid, 210, 211,219	Maltodextrin	Sodium Methyl Cocoyl Taurate
BHA 320, Butylated Hydroxyanisole	MEA -Monoethanolamine	Soy protein concentrate
BHT 321, Butylated Hydroxytoluene	Medilave	Soy protein isolate
Bisphenol-A (BPA)	Mercury	Soy sauce extract
Bouillon and Broth	Methanol	Spices, Seasoning
Brominated vegetable oil (BVO)	Methyl PGME	Splenda
Bronopol anything	Methyl DEGBE, DPGME	Stearalkonium Chloride
Butylcarbamate	Methyl EGPE, EGME, EGEE	Stock
Butylene Glycol	Methylpropane	Succinic acid
Caffeine unless organic & fermented	Mineral Oil	Sucralose
Calcium Caseinate	Miralax	Sugar (chemicalized white processed sugar)
Carbomer	Monoammonium Salt & Carbonate	Sulfites
Carrageenan	Monopotassium Glutamate	Sulphur dioxide
Cationic Surfactants /Ammoniums	Monosodium Glutamate MSG-622	Sunette
Cepacol, ceprim, cepacol chloride	Natrium Glutamate	Sweet 'N Low , Sweet n Safe, Sweet One
Cetafilm, cetamium	Natural beef flavoring	Talc
Cetearehs	Natural Beef or Chicken	Tartrazine 102
Cetrimonium Cloride	Natural chicken flavoring	TEA Triethanolamine Laureth Sulfate
Cetylpyridinium chloride or bromide	Natural flavor(s) & flavoring(s)	Tetrasodium Pyrophoshate (EDTA)
Chloromethylisothiazolin	Natural pork flavoring	Textured Protein
Clorine	Neotame	TBHQ
Coal Tars	Nitrite / Nitrate	Titanium dioxide
Cocoamidopropyl Betaine	NutraSweet	Toluene
Cocoyl Sarcosine	Olestra	Triclosan
DEA- diethanolamine	Paraben (methyl, propyl, butyl, ethyl)	Ultra-pasteurized Soy sauce
Diazolidinyl Urea	Paraffin wax or oil	Urea (Imidazolidinyl)
Dioctyl sodium sulfosuccinate	Partially Hydrogenated veg. oils	Vaseline
Dioxins	Pectin Soy protein	Whey protein concentrate
Disodium Dioctyl Sulfosuccinate	PEG	Whey protein isolate
Disodium Laureth Sulfosuccinate	Petrolatum / jelly	Whey protein Protease
Disodium Oleamide Sulfosuccinate	Phenol	Yeast; Extract, Food, Nutrient
DMDM Hydantoin	Phenylenediamine (PPD)	
Dobendan	Phenylketonuria (PKU)	
EDTA	Phthalates DBP, DMP, DEP	
Enzymes anything Seasonings (the word "seasonings")	Plant Protein Extract	**See LivingAnointed.com to print out a larger copy of this list. Or a smaller cheat sheet listing in color**
Equal	Polyxamer 407	
Ercocet	Polyethylene Gycol (PEG)	

Made in the USA
Charleston, SC
16 November 2014